Medical and Advanced Surgical Management of Pelvic Floor Disorders

Editor

CHERYL B. IGLESIA

OBSTETRICS AND GYNECOLOGY CLINICS OF NORTH AMERICA

www.obgyn.theclinics.com

Consulting Editor
WILLIAM F. RAYBURN

March 2016 • Volume 43 • Number 1

ELSEVIER

1600 John F. Kennedy Boulevard • Suite 1800 • Philadelphia, Pennsylvania, 19103-2899

http://www.theclinics.com

OBSTETRICS AND GYNECOLOGY CLINICS OF NORTH AMERICA Volume 43, Number 1
March 2016 ISSN 0889-8545, ISBN-13: 978-0-323-41655-9

Editor: Kerry Holland
Developmental Editor: Kristen Helm

Obstetrics and Gynecology Clinics (ISSN 0889-8545) is published quarterly by Elsevier Inc., 360 Park Avenue South, New York, NY 10010-1710. Months of issue are March, June, September, and December. Periodicals postage paid at New York, NY, and additional mailing offices. Subscription price per year is $295.00 (US individuals), $597.00 (US institutions), $100.00 (US students), $370.00 (Canadian individuals), $754.00 (Canadian institutions), $225.00 (Canadian students), $450.00 (international individuals), $754.00 (international institutions), and $225.00 (international students). To receive student/resident rate, orders must be accompanied by name of affiliated institution, date of term, and the signature of program/residency coordinator on institution letterhead. Orders will be billed at individual rate until proof of status is received. Foreign air speed delivery is included in all *Clinics* subscription prices. All prices are subject to change without notice. POSTMASTER: Send address changes to *Obstetrics and Gynecology Clinics*, Elsevier Health Sciences Division, Subscription Customer Service, 3251 Riverport Lane, Maryland Heights, MO 63043. **Customer Service: Telephone: 1-800-654-2452 (U.S. and Canada); 314-447-8871 (outside U.S. and Canada). Fax: 314-447-8029. E-mail: journalscustomerservice-usa@elsevier.com (for print support); journalsonlinesupport-usa@elsevier. com (for online support).**

Reprints. For copies of 100 or more of articles in this publication, please contact the Commercial Reprints Department, Elsevier Inc., 360 Park Avenue South, New York, New York 10010-1710. Tel.: 212-633-3874; Fax: 212-633-3820; E-mail: reprints@elsevier.com.

Obstetrics and Gynecology Clinics of North America is also published in Spanish by McGraw-Hill Interamericana Editores S.A., P.O. Box 5-237, 06500, Mexico; in Portuguese by Reichmann and Affonso Editores, Rio de Janeiro, Brazil; and in Greek by Paschalidis Medical Publications, Athens, Greece.

Obstetrics and Gynecology Clinics of North America is covered in MEDLINE/PubMed (Index Medicus), Excerpta Medica, Current Concepts/Clinical Medicine, Science Citation Index, BIOSIS, CINAHL, and ISI/BIOMED.

Contributors

CONSULTING EDITOR

WILLIAM F. RAYBURN, MD, MBA
Associate Dean, Continuing Medical Education and Professional Development, Distinguished Professor and Emeritus Chair, Department of Obstetrics and Gynecology, University of New Mexico School of Medicine, Albuquerque, New Mexico

EDITOR

CHERYL B. IGLESIA, MD, FACOG
Director, Section of Female Pelvic Medicine and Reconstructive Surgery; Professor, Departments of Obstetrics and Gynecology, and Urology, National Center for Advanced Pelvic Surgery, MedStar Washington Hospital Center, Georgetown University School of Medicine, Washington, DC

AUTHORS

PAKEEZA ALAM, MD
Fellow, Female Pelvic Medicine and Reconstructive Surgery, MedStar Washington Hospital Center, Georgetown University, Washington, DC

MATTHEW D. BARBER, MD, MHS
Professor of Surgery, Cleveland Clinic Lerner College of Medicine, Case Western Reserve University; Vice-Chair of Clinical Research, Center for Urogynecology and Reconstructive Pelvic Surgery, Obstetrics, Gynecology and Women's Health Institute, Cleveland Clinic, Cleveland, Ohio

JENNIFER L. HALLOCK, MD
Clinical Fellow, Female Pelvic Medicine and Reconstructive Surgery, Johns Hopkins School of Medicine, Baltimore, Maryland

VICTORIA L. HANDA, MD, MHS
Professor, Gynecology and Obstetrics, Johns Hopkins School of Medicine, Baltimore, Maryland

CHERYL B. IGLESIA, MD, FACOG
Director, Section of Female Pelvic Medicine and Reconstructive Surgery; Professor, Departments of Obstetrics and Gynecology, and Urology, National Center for Advanced Pelvic Surgery, MedStar Washington Hospital Center, Georgetown University School of Medicine, Washington, DC

ERIN SEIFERT LAVELLE, MD
Fellow, Female Pelvic Medicine and Reconstructive Surgery, Department of Obstetrics, Gynecology and Reproductive Sciences, University of Pittsburgh School of Medicine, Pittsburgh, Pennsylvania

PEDRO A. MALDONADO, MD
Clinical Fellow; Assistant Instructor, Division of Female Pelvic Medicine and Reconstructive Surgery, Department of Obstetrics and Gynecology, University of Texas Southwestern Medical Center, Dallas, Texas

ISUZU MEYER, MD
Fellow; Instructor, Division of Urogynecology and Pelvic Reconstructive Surgery, Department of Obstetrics and Gynecology, University of Alabama at Birmingham, Birmingham, Alabama

RACHEL N. PAULS, MD
Program Director; Director of Research, Female Pelvic Medicine and Reconstructive Surgery Fellowship Program, TriHealth Good Samaritan Hospital, Cincinnati, Ohio

LIESCHEN H. QUIROZ, MD
Department of Obstetrics and Gynecology, University of Oklahoma Health Sciences Center, Oklahoma City, Oklahoma

HOLLY E. RICHTER, PhD, MD
Director, Division of Urogynecology and Pelvic Reconstructive Surgery; Professor, Department of Obstetrics and Gynecology, University of Alabama at Birmingham, Birmingham, Alabama

LEE A. RICHTER, MD
Departments of Obstetrics and Gynecology, and Urology, National Center for Advanced Pelvic Surgery, MedStar Washington Hospital Center, Georgetown University School of Medicine, Washington, DC

LAUREN N. SIFF, MD
Fellow, Female Pelvic Medicine and Reconstructive Surgery, Center for Urogynecology and Reconstructive Pelvic Surgery, Obstetrics, Gynecology and Women's Health Institute, Cleveland Clinic, Cleveland, Ohio

ANDREW I. SOKOL, MD
Associate Professor, Departments of Obstetrics and Gynecology, and Urology, National Center for Advanced Pelvic Surgery, MedStar Washington Hospital Center, Georgetown University School of Medicine, Washington, DC

DANIEL E. STONE, MD
Associate Professor, Section of Female Pelvic Medicine and Reconstructive Surgery, Department of Obstetrics and Gynecology, University of Oklahoma Health Sciences Center, Oklahoma City, Oklahoma

CLIFFORD Y. WAI, MD
Associate Professor; Fellowship Director, Division of Female Pelvic Medicine and Reconstructive Surgery, Department of Obstetrics and Gynecology, University of Texas Southwestern Medical Center, Dallas, Texas

EMILY E. WEBER LEBRUN, MD, MS, FACOG
Assistant Professor, Head of Urogynecology, Department of Obstetrics and Gynecology, University of Florida College of Medicine, Gainesville, Florida

NICOLA WHITE, MD
Fellow, Female Pelvic Medicine and Reconstructive Surgery, National Center for Advanced Pelvic Surgery, MedStar Washington Hospital Center, Georgetown University, Washington, DC

JENNIFER YEUNG, DO
Fellow, Female Pelvic Medicine and Reconstructive Surgery, TriHealth Good Samaritan
Hospital, Cincinnati, Ohio

HALINA M. ZYCZYNSKI, MD
Professor and Director, Division of Urogynecology and Pelvic Reconstructive Surgery,
Department of Obstetrics, Gynecology and Reproductive Sciences, University of
Pittsburgh School of Medicine, Pittsburgh, Pennsylvania

Contents

> Using a lifespan model, this article presents new scientific findings regarding risk factors for pelvic floor disorders (PFDs), focusing on the role of childbirth in the development of single or multiple coexisting PFDs. Phase I of the model includes predisposing factors, such as genetic predisposition and race. Phase II includes inciting factors, such as obstetric events. Prolapse, urinary incontinence (UI), and fecal incontinence (FI) are more common among vaginally parous women, although the impact of vaginal delivery on risk of FI is less dramatic than prolapse and UI. Phase III includes intervening factors, such as age and obesity.

> As the field of reconstructive pelvic surgery continues to evolve, with descriptions of new procedures to repair pelvic organ prolapse, it remains imperative to maintain a functional understanding of pelvic floor anatomy and support. The goal of this review is to provide a focused, conceptual approach to differentiating anatomic defects contributing to prolapse in the various compartments of the vagina. Rather than provide exhaustive descriptions of pelvic floor anatomy, basic pelvic floor anatomy is reviewed, new and historical concepts of pelvic floor support are discussed, and relevance to the surgical management of specific anatomic defects is addressed.

> The female vulva is an intricate structure comprising several components. Each structure has been described separately, but the interplay among them and physiologic significance remain controversial. The structures extend inferiorly from the pubic arch and include the mons pubis, labia majora, labia minora, vestibule, and clitoris. The clitoris is widely accepted as the most critical anatomic structure to female sexual arousal and orgasm. The female sexual response cycle is also very complex, requiring emotional and mental stimulation in addition to end organ stimulation.

Fecal incontinence is a highly prevalent and distressing condition that has a negative impact on quality of life. The etiology is often multifactorial, and the evaluation and treatment of this condition can be hindered by a lack of understanding of the mechanisms and currently available treatment options. This article reviews the evidence-based update for the management of fecal incontinence.

Surgical device innovation has been less regulated than drug development, allowing integration of unproven techniques and materials into standard practice. Successful device registries gather information on patient outcomes and can provide postmarket surveillance of new technologies and allow comparison with currently established treatments or devices. The Pelvic Floor Disorders Registry was developed in collaboration with the Food and Drug Administration, device manufacturers, and other stakeholders to serve as a platform for industry-sponsored postmarket device surveillance, investigator-initiated research, and quality and effectiveness benchmarking, all designed to improve the care of women with pelvic floor disorders.

Informed consent is the process in which a patient makes a decision about a surgical procedure or medical intervention after adequate information is relayed by the physician and understood by the patient. This process is critical for reconstructive pelvic surgeries, particularly with the advent of vaginal mesh procedures. In this article, we review the principles of informed consent, the pros and cons of different approaches in reconstructive pelvic surgery, the current legal issues surrounding mesh use for vaginal surgery, and tips on how to incorporate this information when consenting patients for pelvic floor surgery.

This article discusses the background and appraisal of endoluminal ultrasound of the pelvic floor. It provides a detailed anatomic assessment of the muscles and surrounding organs of the pelvic floor. Different anatomic variability and pathology, such as prolapse, fecal incontinence, urinary incontinence, vaginal wall cysts, synthetic implanted material, and pelvic pain, are easily assessed with endoluminal vaginal ultrasound. With pelvic organ prolapse in particular, not only is the prolapse itself seen but the underlying cause related to the anatomic and functional abnormalities of the pelvic floor muscle structures are also visualized.

OBSTETRICS AND GYNECOLOGY CLINICS

THE CLINICS ARE AVAILABLE ONLINE!
Access your subscription at:
www.theclinics.com

Foreword

Keeping Informed About Management Options for Pelvic Floor Disorders

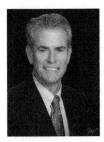

William F. Rayburn, MD, MBA
Consulting Editor

The body of evidence about management of pelvic floor disorders continues to grow in the newly board-certified subspecialty, Female Pelvic Medicine and Reconstructive Surgery. As guest editor, Dr Cheryl Iglesia has organized an excellent issue pertaining to Medical and Advanced Surgical Management of Pelvic Floor Disorders. The latest concepts in anatomy and management options are presented. Common pelvic floor disorders in this issue include pelvic organ prolapse, stress urinary incontinence, overactive bladder, and fecal incontinence.

With the advancing age of the US population, obstetrician-gynecologists are likely to encounter more women with all of these conditions. The range of symptoms resulting from pelvic floor disorders can affect women's physical, psychological, and social well-being and often impose lifestyle restrictions. It is remarkable to me how the severity of symptoms varies from one person to another. Identifying the cause of each woman's symptoms and developing an individualized treatment plan are essential for improving her quality of life. Parity (especially with vaginal birth), menopause, advancing age, prior pelvic surgery, connective tissue disorders, conditions leading to elevated intra-abdominal pressure (eg, obesity, chronic constipation, frequent coughing), and genetic predisposition are examples of contributing factors that come to mind.

Despite the high prevalence of pelvic floor disorders, many women hesitate to seek care or discuss their symptoms with a physician. As a result, many are forced to live with physical, functional, and psychological limitations at home and work. Each person should be evaluated during an office visit to ascertain the nature and severity of the condition resulting in her symptoms. A physical examination is essential to search for confounding or contributing factors. A bimanual examination, including an assessment of pelvic floor muscle strength and voluntary relaxation, is necessary.

Obstet Gynecol Clin N Am 43 (2016) xi–xii
http://dx.doi.org/10.1016/j.ogc.2015.12.002
0889-8545/16/$ – see front matter © 2016 Published by Elsevier Inc.

obgyn.theclinics.com

The screening neurologic examination should include mental status, along with motor and sensory function of the perineum and both lower extremities. Ultrasound imaging of the pelvic floor may be necessary. Articles in this issue nicely describe pelvic ultrasound imaging and review the anatomy of the vulva and female sexual response.

This issue highlights treatment regimens most appropriate when symptoms warrant management. Many patients seek only reassurance or a better understanding if symptoms are mild. Numerous highly effective treatments, supported by recent evidence from randomized controlled trials, are described to manage specific conditions. Treatment options range from conservative to surgical. An important article deals with informed consent for reconstructive pelvic surgery. Alternatives are especially relevant when mesh procedures, whether vaginal or laparoscopic, are being considered. Physicians should assess each woman's goals and expectations for treatment to help her select the best option.

Sexual dysfunction is common among women with pelvic floor disorders. Avoidance of intercourse and other sexual relations is prevalent in affected patients. The extent of sexual dysfunction may be difficult to ascertain because of varied definitions of dysfunction and underreporting of the problem. Therefore, obtaining a sexual history and discussing the impact of their disorder and every treatment option on sexual function are essential.

This issue provides an excellent learning opportunity for the reader to be better equipped when engaging with women with any pelvic floor disorder. Evidence about medical and surgical management options is well presented. I appreciate the authors' expert perspectives in developing a valuable issue in keeping us well-informed.

William F. Rayburn, MD, MBA
Office of Continuing Medical Education
and Professional Development
Department of Obstetrics and Gynecology
University of New Mexico
School of Medicine
MSC 09 5370
1 University of New Mexico
Albuquerque, NM 87131-0001, USA

E-mail address:
wrayburn@salud.unm.edu

Preface

Medical and Advanced Surgical Management of Pelvic Floor Disorders

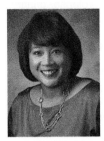

Cheryl B. Iglesia, MD, FACOG
Editor

Female Pelvic Medicine and Reconstructive Surgery is the fourth board-certified subspecialty in Obstetrics and Gynecology and has the added distinction of also being certified by the American Board of Urology. The need for subspecialty services is expected to increase dramatically over the next few decades as the US population grows older and the prevalence of pelvic floor disorders also increases.

In this issue of *Obstetrics and Gynecology Clinics of North America*, experts discuss the latest concepts in the epidemiology, anatomy, and medical and surgical management of pelvic floor disorders. Longitudinal data surrounding the epidemiology of childbirth-related pelvic floor disorders are thoroughly reviewed by Drs Jennifer Hallock and Victoria Handa. Levator ani injury and other predisposing, inciting, and intervening factors are discussed, with a special emphasis on possible future prevention of these disorders. Drs Pedro Maldonado and Clifford Wai discuss new concepts in pelvic floor support and mechanisms of pelvic organ prolapse. Drs Jennifer Yeung and Rachel Pauls outline the latest concepts in the anatomy of female genitalia and the female sexual response. With respect to urinary incontinence, Drs Erin Lavelle and Halina Zyczynski compare the efficacy of treatments for surgical repair of stress urinary incontinence. In another article of this issue, we also include newer treatments for overactive bladder, including β3-agonists and neuromodulation.

Comparative effectiveness of traditional native tissue prolapse repairs is thoroughly reviewed by Drs Lauren Siff and Matthew Barber, while Drs Lee Richter and Andrew Sokol highlight the latest comparative effectiveness trials related to the use of mesh in pelvic organ prolapse repairs. Fecal incontinence is a pelvic floor disorder with a significant negative impact on a woman's quality of life and societal burden. Drs Isuzu Meyer and Holly Richter outline a comprehensive review of available treatment options, including newer technologies. When introducing surgical technologies,

Obstet Gynecol Clin N Am 43 (2016) xiii–xiv
http://dx.doi.org/10.1016/j.ogc.2015.12.001
0889-8545/16/$ – see front matter © 2016 Published by Elsevier Inc.

surveillance on long-term safety and efficacy of these newer modalities remains challenging. Dr Emily Weber LeBrun discusses how registry data can be used to monitor patient-centered and objective outcomes in a variety of prolapse treatments. We also outline some important nuances when consenting for surgical repair of pelvic organ prolapse.

Finally, the use of pelvic floor ultrasonography is one tool for evaluating changes in pelvic floor structures, particularly after mesh implants. Drs Daniel Stone and Lieschen Quiroz describe steps needed to conduct a detailed anatomic assessment of the pelvic floor using endoluminal ultrasound and its applicability for prolapse, urinary and fecal incontinence, and evaluation of complications related to synthetic implanted mesh.

I hope you find this information useful in your clinical practice.

Cheryl B. Iglesia, MD, FACOG
Director, Section of Female Pelvic Medicine
and Reconstructive Surgery
MedStar Washington Hospital Center
Professor, Departments of ObGyn and Urology
Georgetown University School of Medicine
106 Irving Street, Northwest
Suite 405 South
Washington, DC 20010, USA

E-mail address:
cheryl.iglesia@medstar.net

The Epidemiology of Pelvic Floor Disorders and Childbirth: An Update

Jennifer L. Hallock, MD[a], Victoria L. Handa, MD, MHS[b],*

KEYWORDS

- Pelvic floor disorders • Childbirth • Vaginal delivery • Cesarean section
- Urinary incontinence • Pelvic organ prolapse • Fecal incontinence

KEY POINTS

- Pelvic floor disorders are highly prevalent among adult women.
- Vaginal childbirth is strongly associated with the incidence of pelvic floor disorders later in life.
- Injury to the levator ani muscle as well as functional changes in the muscle may result from vaginal birth and may contribute to the development of incontinence and prolapse.
- Prevention and treatment of obesity may reduce the burden of symptomatic pelvic floor disorders.

The study of the epidemiology of any disease starts with case definition. Pelvic floor disorders (PFDs) include stress urinary incontinence (SUI), urgency urinary incontinence (UUI), overactive bladder (OAB), pelvic organ prolapse (POP), and fecal or anal incontinence (FI, AI). Numerous definitions and classification schemes have been proposed for these individual PFDs. Variations in definitions, both in clinical practice and in the literature, create variability in estimates of prevalence and incidence.[1] For instance, mild POP, defined as any degree of prolapse on examination, is practically universal in older women[2]; but women may not have symptoms unless prolapse is more severe.[3] Thus, estimates of the prevalence of POP will be impacted by the threshold used to define the condition.

Additionally, definitions proposed for clinical practice may not be sufficiently precise for epidemiologic research. In 2009, the International Continence Society (ICS) and the

Disclosure statement: This work was supported by R01HD056275 and R01HD082070.
[a] Female Pelvic Medicine & Reconstructive Surgery, Johns Hopkins School of Medicine, 4940 Eastern Avenue, 301 Building, Suite 3200, Baltimore, MD 21224, USA; [b] Gynecology & Obstetrics, Johns Hopkins School of Medicine, 4940 Eastern Avenue, 301 Building, Suite 3200, Baltimore, MD 21224, USA
* Corresponding author.
E-mail address: vhanda1@jhmi.edu

International Urogynecologic Association provided updates on defining PFDs.[4] Urinary incontinence (UI) is defined as involuntary loss of urine. However, the definition does not specify a measurement standard for this condition. Similar limitations are noted with the ICS definitions for other PFDs. OAB is defined as urinary urgency (usually accompanied by frequency and nocturia), with or without UUI, in the absence of urinary tract infection or other obvious pathology. POP is defined as the "descent of one or more of the anterior vaginal wall, posterior vaginal wall, the uterus (cervix) or the apex of the vagina (vaginal vault or cuff scar after hysterectomy)," correlated with symptoms, assisted by any relevant imaging. FI is defined as involuntary loss of feces, whereas AI is involuntary loss of feces or flatus.[4]

As noted by Sung and Hampton in 2009,[1] "the generalized lack of agreement on an epidemiologic definition of incontinence has limited the ability to obtain precise and consistent estimates of prevalence, incidence, and remission rates. In addition, differences in target populations, study and survey methodology, and questionnaire design increase the variability of estimates between studies." Prior publications have addressed various validated standards for the measurement and classification of PFDs.[1,5–7]

PREVALENCE AND PUBLIC HEALTH BURDEN OF PELVIC FLOOR DISORDERS

Despite the challenges of measuring and classifying PFDs in epidemiologic research, recent studies have provided valuable estimates of the prevalence of these conditions. PFDs are common. Based on a cross-sectional study of a nationally representative population of women in the United States, the prevalence of at least one PFD was 23.7%. The prevalence was more than doubled in women 80 years or older.[8] The probability that a woman will undergo surgical correction of POP by 80 years of age is estimated to be 1 in 5.[9,10]

Research also suggests that PFDs often coexist. For example, in a study of more than 5000 parous Swedish women,[11] 46% had at least one disorder and almost a third of these symptomatic women had 2 or more disorders. Similarly, in a Kaiser study, at least one PFD was reported by 34% of women older than 40 years and 16% of symptomatic women had more than one disorder; specifically, 9% of the symptomatic women had both UI and FI and 7% had both UI and POP (**Fig. 1**).[12]

Because of their high prevalence, PFDs have a large economic burden. In 2006, the estimated direct annual cost of ambulatory care for PFDs in the United States was $412 million.[13] As the population ages, health care utilization for PFDs is predicted to grow. Wu and colleagues[14] used US Census Bureau population projections to estimate the total number of women who will undergo surgery for POP from 2010 to 2050 and determined that this number is expected to increase by 48.2% over these 4 decades.

The limitation of studies on health care utilization is that some women with PFDs do not seek care. In a population-based sample of women 40 years or older, the prevalence of UI was 41%; but only 25% of symptomatic women sought care, 23% received some care, and 12% received subspecialty care.[15] In a community-based Internet survey of women older than 45 years, 19% reported accidental bowel leakage but only 29% of those had sought care.[16] Thus, the incidence of care seeking provides an underestimate of the public health burden of PFDs among US women.

PELVIC FLOOR DISORDERS AS CHRONIC DISEASE

One model for conceptualizing the development of PFDs in women was published in 1998 by Bump and Norton[17] (**Fig. 2**). This model provides a framework for discussion

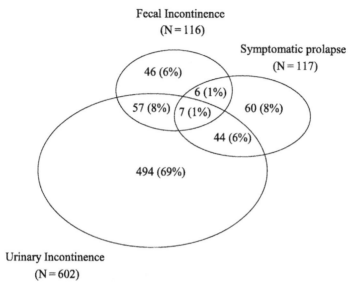

Fig. 1. Overlap of the prevalence of UI (weekly or more), symptomatic POP, and FI (leaking monthly or more) in 714 symptomatic women. (*From* Rortveit G, Subak LL, Thom DH, et al. Urinary incontinence, fecal incontinence and pelvic organ prolapse in a population-based, racially diverse cohort. Female Pelvic Med Reconstr Surg 2010;16(5):280; with permission.)

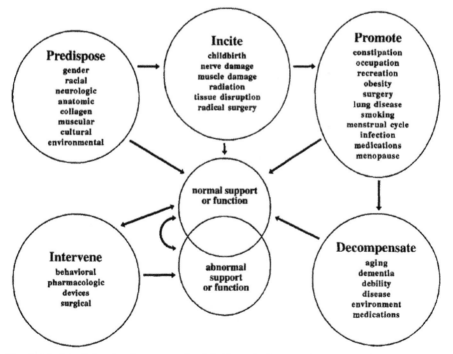

Fig. 2. Model of the development of pelvic floor dysfunction in women. (*From* Bump RC, Norton P. Epidemiology and natural history of pelvic floor dysfunction. Obstet Gynecol Clin North Am 1998;25(4):734; with permission.)

of the progression from normal to abnormal pelvic support and pelvic organ function, organizing risk factors into categories: intervening, predisposing, inciting, promoting, and decompensating. As others have observed,[1] this model may not explain an individual's progression of disease and it does not provide an indication of the burden of one risk factor compared with others.

Another way of conceptualizing the epidemiology of PFDs is a model that takes into account the chronic nature of the disorders. The life course or lifespan approach is a theory used for chronic disease epidemiology.[18] The key concepts include the study of the disease process during gestation, childhood, adolescence, young adulthood, and later adult life, within the individual's life course and across generations. The model emphasizes the temporal relationship between exposure variables and their interrelationships.

The lifespan approach can be used for reproductive health.[19] In 2008, DeLancey and colleagues[20] proposed the Lifespan Model for Pelvic Floor Disorders (**Fig. 3**). Three phases were explored: phase I for predisposing factors, such as growth and development; phase II for inciting factors, such as birth-induced changes; and finally phase III for intervening factors, such as age-related changes or lifestyle factors. It seems reasonable that the lifespan approach can be used to further characterize known and suspected risk factors for PFDs.

Two methods of using the lifespan theory are the critical period method and the accumulation of risk method. The latter can be further categorized based on whether individual risk factors (1) act separately, (2) cluster together, (3) accumulate in an additive fashion (known as a chain of risk), or (4) have a final trigger effect risk factor. Accumulation of risk may be most appropriate for modeling PFD epidemiology. For instance, Memon and Handa[21] provided a graphical display of obstetric exposures in a population of primiparous women who delivered vaginally (**Fig. 4**).[21] As **Fig. 4** shows, these obstetric exposures are clustered and have considerable overlap. Using a lifespan model with an accumulation of risk framework, the sections that follow present a perspective on new scientific findings regarding risk factors for PFDs.

PHASE I: PREDISPOSING FACTORS FOR PELVIC FLOOR DISORDERS
Genetic Predisposition

A genetic cause for PFDs has not been identified, although epidemiologic evidence for a genetic predisposition accumulates. For example, a meta-analysis of clinical studies

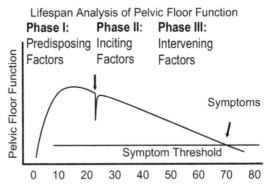

Fig. 3. The lifespan model of pelvic floor function. This graph shows the development of PFDs across 3 phases of a woman's life. (*From* DeLancey JOL, Low LK, Miller JM, et al. Graphic integration of causal factors of pelvic floor disorders: an integrated lifespan model. Am J Obstet Gynecol 2008;199:610.e2; with permission.)

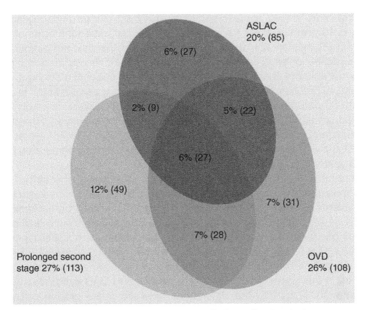

Fig. 4. Clustering of obstetric exposures in a population of 418 primiparous women who delivered vaginally. ASLAC, anal sphincter laceration; OVD, operative vaginal delivery. (*From* Memon HU, Handa VL. Vaginal childbirth and pelvic floor disorders. Womens Health (Lond Engl) 2013;9(3):267; with permission.)

on family history of POP calculated that the relative odds for POP among women with a genetic predisposition was 2.58.[22] A meta-analysis provided moderate evidence of the genetic association for urinary symptoms in women, with certain genes having an odds ratio (OR) of 2.5 for OAB and 2.1 for SUI.[23] Although specific genetic predisposition has not been identified, a systematic review of genetic studies found that collagen type 3 alpha 1 was associated with POP (OR 4.79).[24]

Race

Some studies suggest that the prevalence of prolapse and incontinence are associated with race. For example, Kaiser investigators found that Latina and white women had a higher risk of symptomatic POP than African American women (prevalence ratio 4.89 and 5.35, respectively).[25] In a related Kaiser study, the age-adjusted prevalence of weekly UI was significantly different among Hispanic (36%), white (30%), African American (25%), and Asian American (19%) women (*P*>.001).[26] However, other studies have not found significant racial differences in UI.[8,27] Also, FI does not seem to be associated with race.[28] It is worth noting that studies based on symptoms reported by women of different race may be biased by culture-based differences in perceptions of symptoms.[29]

PHASE II: INCITING FACTORS FOR PELVIC FLOOR DISORDERS

The second phase of the lifespan model focuses on the impact of acquired risk factors, such as obstetric events.

Severe and symptomatic POP is much more common in vaginally parous versus nulliparous women.[30–32] Among multiparous women, the increase is most dramatic with the first birth.[30,31] In a cross-sectional study by Quiroz and colleagues[30] of women aged 40 years or older, vaginal delivery (VD) increased the odds of prolapse to or beyond the hymen (OR 9.73), but an additional VD was not associated with increased odds. In contrast, cesarean delivery (CD) was not associated with prolapse. Two additional epidemiologic studies of parous women suggest a strong association between vaginal (vs cesarean) delivery on the odds of prolapse later in life. In a study of more than 1000 parous women 5 to 10 years from a first delivery, a history of one or more vaginal births was strongly associated with POP to or beyond the hymen on physical examination (OR 5.6, 95% confidence interval [CI] 2.2–14.7).[31] An association between VD and prolapse symptoms was also observed among primiparous Swedish women (20 years after one VD or CD).[32]

UI, most notably SUI, is also strongly associated with vaginal childbirth.[31,33,34] In a Swedish population of women 20 years from a single delivery, VD was associated with higher UI severity (adjusted OR 1.68, 95% CI 1.40–2.03) and UI bother (adjusted OR 1.85, 95% CI 1.42–2.39).[34] In a cohort of women 5 to 10 years from first delivery,[31] a history of one or more vaginal births was associated with significantly greater odds of SUI (OR 2.9, 95% CI 1.5–5.5) but not OAB (OR 1.7, 95% CI 0.8–3.5). The impact of vaginal birth on UI is most notable in the immediate postpartum period. For example, in this same cohort study, severe SUI and OAB symptoms were more common after VD than CD; but differences between these groups decreased as time since childbirth increased.[33]

FI also seems to be more common among vaginally parous women, although the impact of VD on risk of FI is less dramatic than for other PFDs. Using data from the Nurses' Health Study, Townsend and colleagues[35] reported that the odds of liquid FI increased with each pregnancy beginning with the first (OR 1.29, 1.66, 1.75, 1.74, and 1.84 for 1, 2, 3, 4, and 5 or more pregnancies, respectively). The investigators hypothesized a cumulative effect of multiple births on global pelvic floor dysfunction. However, other studies have suggested that VD (in the absence of a recognized sphincter laceration) does not seem to increase the risk of AI compared with CD.[36]

Labor, in the absence of VD, does not seem to modify the later development of PFDs. Among women who have delivered exclusively by cesarean (ie, across all their births), the risk of PFD does not seem to be increased by a history of active labor or complete cervical dilation before CD.[31] In contrast, operative vaginal birth seems to be a powerful risk factor for the development of PFDs. Compared with uninstrumented VD, operative delivery (by forceps or vacuum) significantly increases the odds for all PFDs, with the highest increase for POP (OR 7.5, 95% CI 2.7–20.9).[31]

Unfortunately, in some studies the impact of childbirth on the later incidence of PFDs may be influenced by recall bias. For instance, one study of parous women suggested that women with symptoms of PFDs were more likely to report a history of anal sphincter laceration, even if the medical record did not confirm a laceration ($P = .025$).[37] Thus, studies that rely on participant recall may not accurately reflect the association between obstetric events and development of PFDs.

Given the strong accumulating evidence of an association between vaginal birth and PFDs, it is important to identify pathophysiologic mechanisms for the observed association. One potential mechanism may be damage to the levator ani muscle (LAM). The work of Delancey[38–40] and Dietz and colleagues[41–43] has done much to draw attention to the role of levator tears in the development of PFDs. The LAM can be injured by stretch (overdistension, or microtrauma) or avulsion (disruption of the muscle, or macrotrauma).[44] In a review by Schwertner-Tiepelmann and colleagues,[45] the prevalence of LAM injuries was 13% to 36% in vaginally parous women.

However, the prognosis after levator injury is uncertain. Imaging suggests that levator injury may resolve over time.[46,47] Van Delft and colleagues[48] found that most levator avulsions diagnosed at 3 months post partum were not evident at 12 months (62%, 95% CI 41%–79%). Of 30 levator avulsions, 9 were persistent. Women with persistent evidence of avulsion were more likely to have symptoms of PFD and weakened pelvic floor muscle strength. Although both levator avulsion and overdistension have been associated with reduced contractile function,[44] the fact that women with levator ani defects are still able to contract the pelvic floor muscles may provide evidence that perhaps noninjured muscles are compensating for injured muscles.[49]

Even in the absence of levator injury, levator muscle dynamics may be impacted by childbirth. On ultrasound, the number of vaginal births has been associated with increased hiatal area ($P<.001$); the effect is most pronounced after the first vaginal birth.[50] Changes in the levator hiatus are also more likely to persist after VD than after prelabor CD.[51] However, regardless of delivery route, the levator hiatus remains more distensible after delivery compared with measurements at 12 weeks' gestation.[51] Additionally, changes in the appearance of vaginal fornices on MR imaging has been observed after delivery[52]; this suggests a possible role of paravaginal injury during delivery on subsequent development of anterior vaginal wall prolapse.

As more information emerges about the incidence of levator injury, a critical question is whether this obstetric complication leads to PFDs. In a study of women delivered by operative vaginal birth, LAM avulsion observed on 3-dimensional (3D) transperineal ultrasound was associated with symptoms of prolapse ($P = .036$) but not objective evidence of prolapse ($P = .20$).[53] Others have found that objective evidence of prolapse is more common among those with LAM injury.[43] For example, among primiparous women 12 months after delivery,[54] levator avulsion was associated with objective and subjective measures of POP (OR 4.8, 95% CI 1.99–11.34).

Levator injury has been associated with persistent enlargement of the levator hiatus,[48] which may plausibly contribute to the development of prolapse. For example, the size of the genital hiatus on physical examination (a proxy for the size of the levator hiatus[55,56]) is a predictor of worsening pelvic organ support over time.[57] Specifically, the odds for worsening support over 12 to 18 months seems to be doubled among women with a genital hiatus greater than or equal to 2 compared with those with a smaller genital hiatus (OR 2.36, 95% CI 1.03–5.43). In another study, women with de novo SUI 2 days postpartum had higher levator hiatus transverse diameter and area ($P<.05$).[58] This finding suggests that the size of the levator hiatus may be a risk factor for the development of PFDs.

Mechanism of Injury

In a 3D computer model created from digitized cadaveric anatomy, investigators determined that the nerves to the anal sphincter stretched during VD, beyond the 15% threshold known to cause permanent damage in appendicular peripheral nerves.[59] This model showed that greater nerve strain occurred if the nerve fixation point was more proximal. The inferior rectal branch was the most strained (35%), followed by the perineal nerve branch innervating the anal sphincter (33%), then the branches to the posterior labia (15%) and urethral sphincter (13%). Thus, neuropraxia is likely after vaginal birth; but the impact on the later development of PFDs is not currently known.

Among women who deliver vaginally, maternal and fetal factors may influence the probability of levator trauma and other obstetric sequelae. One obvious fetal factor is birth weight. Birth weight seems to be a risk factor for symptomatic POP.[32] In one study of Swedish women (assessed by mailed symptom questionnaire), symptomatic POP increased by 3% (OR 1.03; 95% CI 1.02–1.05) for each 100-g increase of infant weight. Short mothers who were 160 cm or less and who delivered a child weighting 4000 g or more had a doubled prevalence of symptomatic POP compared with short mothers with smaller babies (OR 2.06; 95% CI 1.19–3.55).

The probability of obstetric neuromuscular injuries may also be influenced by antepartum accommodation to childbirth. In a recent editorial, Nygaard[60] proposed a "bendy person toy" analogy for vaginal childbirth.[60] She proposed that the pelvic floor is a dynamic structure that changes to accommodate the fetal head. For instance, it has been shown that the levator hiatus enlarges during pregnancy.[51] Recent studies using rat models found that, predelivery, there was a 21% to 37% increase in pelvic floor muscle fiber length,[61] as additional sarcomeres were added and collagen synthesis increased in intramuscular extracellular matrix.[62] Women who experience less levator enlargement may possibly be predisposed to injury; smaller levator hiatal dimensions with voluntary contraction have been associated with subsequent operative VD or CD.[63] Additionally, greater first-trimester elastase activity has been associated with uncomplicated spontaneous VD.[61] Differences in adaptation during late pregnancy might contribute to differences among women with respect to progress during labor and the occurrence of soft tissue trauma with VD.

PHASE III: INTERVENING FACTORS FOR PELVIC FLOOR DISORDERS
Age

Age is known to be associated with the prevalence and severity for all PFDs. For example, in a population-based cross-sectional study, Miedel and colleagues[64] asked 5489 women aged 30 to 79 years with an intact uterus and no prior pelvic surgery to complete a survey using validated questionnaires for symptomatic POP. They found age had an independent significant association with symptomatic prolapse. Age was also an independent risk factor for FI among participants in the US National Health and Nutrition Examination Survey 2005 to 2010.[28] Prevalence increased from 2.91% among 20- to 29-year-old participants, to 16.16% among participants aged 70 years and older. Similarly, in the Nurses' Health Study, the reported prevalence of liquid or solid stool incontinence at least monthly increased from 9% in women aged 62 to 64 years to 17% in women aged 85 to 87 years.[65]

Obesity

Obesity seems to be a risk factor for symptoms of prolapse,[32,66] although an association with objective measures of prolapse is less clear. For example, in the SWEPOP (Swedish Pregnancy, Obesity and Pelvic floor) study,[32] symptomatic POP increased 3% with each unit increase of current body mass index (OR 1.03; 95% CI 1.01–1.05). Unfortunately, there was no objective measure of prolapse severity in this study. In a clinical trial of a weight-loss program,[66] symptoms of POP were recorded for 338 women at baseline and 6 months after a weight loss or educational program. At baseline, a higher proportion of obese women reported feeling vaginal bulging compared with overweight women (13% vs 0%, $P<.01$); of the obese women, 9% reported bothersome sensation of vaginal bulge. Unfortunately, at 6 months, there were no significant differences in improvement of self-reported bothersome prolapse symptoms in women in the weight loss or the control group.

There is increasing evidence that obesity is a strong risk factor for the incidence and progression of UI and AI.[33] In a mailed questionnaire to women contemplating bariatric surgery, Chen and colleagues[67] determined that obese women had a fourfold risk of UI and twofold risk of AI compared with nonobese controls. The prevalence of at least one PFD was 75% in the obese group, compared with 44% of the nonobese (*P*<.0001). In a longitudinal cohort study of parous women, obese women experienced a significantly greater increase in UI bother over time, compared with nonobese women.[33] Thus, obesity is not only a risk factor for incontinence but also seems to accelerate incontinence progression over time.

Fortunately, either diet/exercise or bariatric surgery can reduce UI. The investigators of the Longitudinal Assessment of Bariatric Surgery 2 recently published their 3-year follow-up data.[68] Prevalent UI, defined as at least weekly UI episodes, was 49.3% at baseline in the women, 18.3% at 1 year (mean weight loss 29.5%), and 24.8% at 3 years. Similar optimistic findings were reported by the investigators of the Program to Reduce Incontinence by Diet and Exercise, even with modest weight loss defined as 5% to 10% of body weight.[69] Compared with a reference of participants who gained weight, the women who lost 5% to 10% of their body weight were significantly more likely to experience a reduction in UI episodes and were more likely to achieve at least a 70% reduction in the frequency of total UI and urge UI episodes. Similarly, women with liquid stool FI who lost at least 5 kg and/or increased their dietary fiber intake had reduced FI frequency (*P* = .001 and *P* = .05, respectively) at up to 18 months follow-up.[70]

SUMMARY

The lifespan approach provides a conceptual framework for the interaction of causal factors for PFDs over time.[20] This framework is particularly useful for understanding the role of childbirth, and VD in particular, in the development of single or multiple coexisting PFDs. The complex interactions between pregnancy physiology, childbirth mechanics, obstetric interventions, and predisposing factors (such as genetics) are still unclear. For instance, although cesarean birth is associated with a lower incidence of PFDs later in life, cesarean section without labor does not completely protect a woman from developing PFDs[31]; moreover, although PFDs are highly prevalent among vaginally parous women, severe PFDs are not universal among such women.

Recent studies have shown that the pelvic floor is a dynamic structure that adapts during pregnancy and delivery by expanding the levator hiatus, increasing elastase activity, and lengthening pelvic floor muscle fibers. Future studies with animal or imaging models will provide even more insight into these mechanics. Although the impact of childbirth on the development of PFDs is clear, other inciting and intervening factors play a critical role. Fortunately, not all women with obstetric risk factors develop symptomatic PFDs. Some remain asymptomatic, others experience transient symptoms, and yet others develop significant symptoms much later in life. Antenatal prediction of pelvic floor injury is not currently feasible.[71,72] At the current time, the prevention and treatment of obesity is an important component to PFD prevention. Other proposed primary and secondary prevention strategies (such as elective cesarean section[73,74]) may be based on insufficient evidence; recommendations for intervention based on perceived risk should be balanced against risks and costs.

REFERENCES

1. Sung VW, Hampton BS. Epidemiology of pelvic floor dysfunction. Obstet Gynecol Clin North Am 2009;36(3):421–43.
2. Nygaard I, Bradley C, Brandt D. Pelvic organ prolapse in older women: prevalence and risk factors. Obstet Gynecol 2004;104(3):489–97.
3. Gutman RE, Ford DE, Quiroz LH, et al. Is there a pelvic organ prolapse threshold that predicts pelvic floor symptoms? Am J Obstet Gynecol 2008;199(6):683.e1–7.

4. Haylen B, de Ridder D, Freeman RM, et al. An International Urogynecological Association (IUGA)/International Continence Society (ICS) Joint Report on the terminology for female pelvic floor dysfunction. Neurourol Urodyn 2010;29:4–20.
5. Madoff RD, Parker SC, Varma MG, et al. Faecal incontinence in adults. Lancet 2004;364(9434):621–32.
6. Jelovsek JE, Maher C, Barber MD. Pelvic organ prolapse. Lancet 2007; 369(9566):1027–38.
7. Barber MD. Questionnaires for women with pelvic floor disorders. Int Urogynecol J 2006;18(4):461–5.
8. Nygaard I, Barber MD. Prevalence of symptomatic pelvic floor disorders in US women. JAMA 2008;300(11):1311–6.
9. Wu JM, Matthews CA, Conover MM, et al. Lifetime risk of stress urinary incontinence or pelvic organ prolapse surgery. Obstet Gynecol 2014;123(6):1201–6.
10. Smith FJ, Holman CDJ, Moorin RE, et al. Lifetime risk of undergoing surgery for pelvic organ prolapse. Obstet Gynecol 2010;116(5):1096–100.
11. Gyhagen M, Åkervall S, Milsom I. Clustering of pelvic floor disorders 20 years after one vaginal or one cesarean birth. Int Urogynecol J 2015;26(8):1115–21.
12. Rortveit G, Subak LL, Thom DH, et al. Urinary incontinence, fecal incontinence and pelvic organ prolapse in a population-based, racially diverse cohort. Female Pelvic Med Reconstr Surg 2010;16(5):278–83.
13. Sung VW, Washington B, Raker CA. Costs of ambulatory care related to female pelvic floor disorders in the United States. Am J Obstet Gynecol 2010;202(5): 483.e1–4.
14. Wu JM, Kawasaki A, Hundley AF, et al. Predicting the number of women who will undergo incontinence and prolapse surgery, 2010 to 2050. Am J Obstet Gynecol 2011;205(3):230.e1–5.
15. Minassian VA, Yan XS, Lichtenfeld MJ, et al. The iceberg of health care utilization in women with urinary incontinence. Int Urogynecol J 2012;23(8):1087–93.
16. Brown HW, Wexner SD, Lukacz ES. Factors associated with care seeking among women with accidental bowel leakage. Female Pelvic Med Reconstr Surg 2013; 19(2):66–71.
17. Bump RC, Norton P. Epidemiology and natural history of pelvic floor dysfunction. Obstet Gynecol Clin North Am 1998;25(4):723–46.
18. Ben-Shlomo Y, Kuh D. A life course approach to chronic disease epidemiology: conceptual models, empirical challenges and interdisciplinary perspectives. Int J Epidemiol 2002;31:285–93.
19. Mishra GD, Cooper R, Kuh D. A life course approach to reproductive health: theory and methods. Maturitas 2010;65(2):92–7.
20. DeLancey JOL, Low LK, Miller JM, et al. Graphic integration of causal factors of pelvic floor disorders: an integrated life span model. Am J Obstet Gynecol 2008; 199:610.e1–5.
21. Memon HU, Handa VL. Vaginal childbirth and pelvic floor disorders. Womens Health (Lond Engl) 2013;9(3):265–77.
22. Lince SL, van Kempen LC, Vierhout ME, et al. A systematic review of clinical studies on hereditary factors in pelvic organ prolapse. Int Urogynecol J 2012; 23(10):1327–36.
23. Cartwright R, Mangera A, Tikkinen KAO, et al. Systematic review and meta-analysis of candidate gene association studies of lower urinary tract symptoms in men. Eur Urol 2014;66(4):752–68.
24. Ward RM, Velez Edwards DR, Edwards T, et al. Genetic epidemiology of pelvic organ prolapse: a systematic review. Am J Obstet Gynecol 2014;211(4):326–35.

25. Whitcomb EL, Rortveit G, Brown JS, et al. Racial differences in pelvic organ prolapse. Obstet Gynecol 2009;114(6):1271–7.
26. Thom DH, Van Den Eeden SK, Ragins AI, et al. Differences in prevalence of urinary incontinence by race/ethnicity. J Urol 2006;175(1):259–64.
27. Waetjen LE, Xing G, Johnson WO, et al. Factors associated with seeking treatment for urinary incontinence during the menopausal transition. Obstet Gynecol 2015;125(5):1071–9.
28. Ditah I, Devaki P, Luma HN, et al. Prevalence, trends, and risk factors for fecal incontinence in United States adults, 2005-2010. Clin Gastroenterol Hepatol 2014;12(4):636–43.e2.
29. Maserejian NN, Chen S, Chiu GR, et al. Treatment status and progression or regression of lower urinary tract symptoms in a general adult population sample. J Urol 2014;191(1):107–13.
30. Quiroz L, Muñoz A, Shippey SH, et al. Vaginal parity and pelvic organ prolapse. J Reprod Med 2011;55(3–4):93–8.
31. Handa VL, Blomquist JL, Knoepp LR, et al. Pelvic floor disorders 5-10 years after vaginal or cesarean childbirth. Obstet Gynecol 2011;118(4):777–84.
32. Gyhagen M, Bullarbo M, Nielsen TF, et al. Prevalence and risk factors for pelvic organ prolapse 20 years after childbirth: a national cohort study in singleton primiparae after vaginal or caesarean delivery. BJOG 2012;120(2):152–60.
33. Handa VL, Pierce CB, Muñoz A, et al. Longitudinal changes in overactive bladder and stress incontinence among parous women. Neurourol Urodyn 2014;34(4):356–61.
34. Gyhagen M, Bullarbo M, Nielsen TF, et al. A comparison of the long-term consequences of vaginal delivery versus caesarean section on the prevalence, severity and bothersomeness of urinary incontinence subtypes: a national cohort study in primiparous women. BJOG 2013;120:1548–55.
35. Townsend MK, Matthews CA, Whitehead WE, et al. Risk factors for fecal incontinence in older women. Am J Gastroenterol 2013;108(1):113–9.
36. Evers EC, Blomquist JL, McDermott KC, et al. Obstetrical anal sphincter laceration and anal incontinence 5-10 years after childbirth. Am J Obstet Gynecol 2012;207(5):425.e1–6.
37. Chen C, Smith LJ, Pierce CB, et al. Do symptoms of pelvic floor disorders bias maternal recall of obstetrical events up to 10 years after delivery? Female Pelvic Med Reconstr Surg 2015;21(3):129–34.
38. Strohbehn K, Ellis JH, Strohbehn JA, et al. Magnetic resonance imaging of the levator ani with anatomic correlation. Obstet Gynecol 1996;87:277–85.
39. DeLancey JOL, Kearney R, Chou Q, et al. The appearance of levator ani muscle abnormalities in magnetic resonance images after vaginal delivery. Obstet Gynecol 2003;101:46–53.
40. Ashton-Miller JA, DeLancey JOL. On the biomechanics of vaginal birth and common sequelae. Annu Rev Biomed Eng 2009;11(1):163–76.
41. Dietz HP, Wilson PD. Childbirth and pelvic floor trauma. Best Pract Res Clin Obstet Gynaecol 2005;19(6):913–24.
42. Dietz HP, Lanzarone V. Levator trauma after vaginal delivery. Obstet Gynecol 2005;106:707–12.
43. Dietz HP, Simpson JM. Levator trauma is associated with pelvic organ prolapse. BJOG 2008;115(8):979–84.
44. Guzmán Rojas R, Wong V, Shek KL, et al. Impact of levator trauma on pelvic floor muscle function. Int Urogynecol J 2013;25(3):375–80.

45. Schwertner-Tiepelmann N, Thakar R, Sultan AH, et al. Obstetric levator ani muscle injuries: current status. Ultrasound Obstet Gynecol 2012;39(4):372–83.
46. Stær-Jensen J, Siafarikas F, Hilde G, et al. Postpartum recovery of levator hiatus and bladder neck mobility in relation to pregnancy. Obstet Gynecol 2015;125(3): 531–9.
47. Miller JM, Low LK, Zielinski R, et al. Evaluating maternal recovery from labor and delivery: bone and levator ani injuries. Am J Obstet Gynecol 2015;213(2): 188.e1–11.
48. van Delft K, Thakar R, Sultan AH, et al. The natural history of levator avulsion one year following childbirth: a prospective study. BJOG 2014;122:1266–73.
49. Hilde G, Staer-Jensen J, Siafarikas F, et al. How well can pelvic floor muscles with major defects contract? A cross-sectional comparative study 6 weeks after delivery using transperineal 3D/4D ultrasound and manometer. BJOG 2013;120(11):1423–9.
50. Atan IK, Gerges B, Shek KL, et al. The association between vaginal parity and hiatal dimensions: a retrospective observational study in a tertiary urogynaecological centre. BJOG 2014;122(6):867–72.
51. van Veelen GA, Schweitzer KJ, van der Vaart CH. Ultrasound imaging of the pelvic floor: changes in anatomy during and after first pregnancy. Ultrasound Obstet Gynecol 2014;44(4):476–80.
52. Cassadó-Garriga J, Wong V, Shek K, et al. Can we identify changes in fascial paravaginal supports after childbirth? Aust N Z J Obstet Gynaecol 2014;55(1):70–5.
53. Memon HU, Blomquist JL, Dietz HP, et al. Comparison of levator ani muscle avulsion injury after forceps-assisted and vacuum-assisted vaginal childbirth. Obstet Gynecol 2015;125(5):1080–7.
54. Durnea CM, Khashan AS, Kenny LC, et al. Prevalence, etiology and risk factors of pelvic organ prolapse in premenopausal primiparous women. Int Urogynecol J 2014;25(11):1463–70.
55. Dietz HP, Shek C, De Leon J, et al. Ballooning of the levator hiatus. Ultrasound Obstet Gynecol 2008;31(6):676–80.
56. Khunda A, Shek KL, Dietz HP. Can ballooning of the levator hiatus be determined clinically? Am J Obstet Gynecol 2012;206(3):246.e1–4.
57. Pierce CB, Hallock JL, Blomquist JL, et al. Longitudinal changes in pelvic organ support among parous women. Female Pelvic Med Reconstr Surg 2012;18(4): 227–32.
58. Falkert A, Endress E, Weigl M, et al. Three-dimensional ultrasound of the pelvic floor 2 days after first delivery: influence of constitutional and obstetric factors. Ultrasound Obstet Gynecol 2010;35(5):583–8.
59. Lien K-C, Morgan DM, DeLancey JOL, et al. Pudendal nerve stretch during vaginal birth: a 3D computer simulation. Am J Obstet Gynecol 2005;192(5): 1669–76.
60. Nygaard I. New directions in understanding how the pelvic floor prepares for and recovers from vaginal delivery. Am J Obstet Gynecol 2015;213(2):121–2.
61. Oliphant SS, Nygaard IE, Zong W, et al. Maternal adaptations in preparation for parturition predict uncomplicated spontaneous delivery outcome. Am J Obstet Gynecol 2014;211(6):630.e1–7.
62. Alperin M, Lawley DM, Esparza MC, et al. Pregnancy-induced adaptations in the intrinsic structure of rat pelvic floor muscles. Am J Obstet Gynecol 2015;213(2): 191.e1–7.
63. van Veelen GA, Schweitzer KJ, van Hoogenhuijze NE, et al. Association between levator hiatal dimensions on ultrasound during first pregnancy and mode of delivery. Ultrasound Obstet Gynecol 2015;45(3):333–8.

64. Miedel A, Tegerstedt G, Moehle-Schmidt M, et al. Nonobstetric risk factors for symptomatic pelvic organ prolapse. Obstet Gynecol 2009;113:1089–97.
65. Townsend MK, Matthews CA, Whitehead WE, et al. Risk factors for fecal incontinence in older women. Am J Gastroenterol 2012;108(1):113–9.
66. Myers DL, Sung VW, Richter HE, et al. Prolapse symptoms in overweight and obese women before and after weight loss. Female Pelvic Med Reconstr Surg 2012;18(1):55–9.
67. Chen CCG, Gatmaitan P, Koepp S, et al. Obesity is associated with increased prevalence and severity of pelvic floor disorders in women considering bariatric surgery. Surg Obes Relat Dis 2015;5(4):411–5.
68. Subak LL, King WC, Belle SH, et al. Urinary incontinence before and after bariatric surgery. JAMA Intern Med 2015;175(8):1378–87.
69. Wing RR, Creasman JM, West DS, et al. Improving urinary incontinence in overweight and obese women through modest weight loss. Obstet Gynecol 2010;116(2 Part 1):284–92.
70. Markland AD, Richter HE, Burgio KL, et al. Weight loss improves fecal incontinence severity in overweight and obese women with urinary incontinence. Int Urogynecol J 2011;22(9):1151–7.
71. van Delft K, Thakar R, Sultan AH, et al. Levator ani muscle avulsion during childbirth: a risk prediction model. BJOG 2014;121(9):1155–63.
72. Lavy Y, Sand PK, Kaniel CI, et al. Can pelvic floor injury secondary to delivery be prevented? Int Urogynecol J 2011;23(2):165–73.
73. Koc O, Duran B. Role of elective cesarean section in prevention of pelvic floor disorders. Curr Opin Obstet Gynecol 2012;24(5):318–23.
74. Wilson D, Dornan J, Milsom I, et al. UR-CHOICE: can we provide mothers-to-be with information about the risk of future pelvic floor dysfunction? Int Urogynecol J 2014;25(11):1449–52.

Pelvic Organ Prolapse
New Concepts in Pelvic Floor Anatomy

 CrossMark

Pedro A. Maldonado, MD*, Clifford Y. Wai, MD

KEYWORDS

- Prolapse • Anatomy • Pelvic floor • Compartments • Concepts • Theories

KEY POINTS

- A conceptual understanding of pelvic floor anatomy is essential for surgeons in managing prolapse of the anterior, posterior, and apical compartments of the vagina.
- The emerging concept of cervical elongation is important in the evaluation of apical compartment prolapse.
- The development of anterior and apical compartment prolapse appears intimately associated, as demonstrated by 3-dimensional models.
- Dynamic magnetic resonance defecography may help objectively identify posterior compartment defects not easily seen on physical examination and evaluate symptoms of dysfunctional emptying.

INTRODUCTION

Our knowledge of pelvic floor dysfunction can be greatly enhanced through a better appreciation and knowledge of the anatomic principles that define pelvic floor support in women. As the field of reconstructive pelvic surgery continues to evolve, with the increasing incorporation of mesh for the repair of pelvic organ prolapse, it remains imperative to maintain a functional and fundamental understanding of pelvic floor anatomy. The goal of this review was to provide a focused, conceptual approach to differentiating anatomic defects contributing to prolapse in the various compartments of the vagina. Rather than provide exhaustive anatomic descriptions, basic pelvic floor anatomy is reviewed, new and historical concepts of pelvic floor support are discussed, and relevance to the surgical management of specific anatomic defects is addressed.

Disclosure Statement: The authors have nothing to disclose.
Division of Female Pelvic Medicine and Reconstructive Surgery, Department of Obstetrics and Gynecology, University of Texas Southwestern Medical Center, Dallas, TX, USA
* Corresponding author. Department of Obstetrics and Gynecology, 5323 Harry Hines Boulevard, G6.220, Dallas, TX 75390-9032.
E-mail address: pedro.maldonado@utsouthwestern.edu

FUNDAMENTALS OF PELVIC ANATOMY

Advanced knowledge and conceptual understanding of pelvic floor anatomy and support are essential in guiding surgeons in the surgical management of prolapse of the anterior, posterior, and apical compartments of the vagina. Pelvic floor support is defined, in large part, by the complex and dynamic interactions of the muscles and connective tissue attachments within the bony pelvis.

In general, the bony pelvis consists of 4 major components: bilateral hip bones (ilium, ischium, and pubis), the sacrum, and the coccyx. The ilium, ischium, and pubis are fused at the cup-shaped acetabulum, articulating with the femoral head. The pelvic halves are joined at the sacroiliac joints (synovial) posteriorly and the symphysis pubis (cartilaginous) anteriorly. The pelvis is artificially divided into a "true" and the "false" pelvis. The *false pelvis* is located superior to the iliopectineal line, coursing along the superior edge of the superior pubic ramus, and circumferentially forms what is termed the pelvic brim. More relevant to pelvic floor support is the *true pelvis*, which is located below the pelvic brim. Within the true pelvis are the sacrotuberous and sacrospinous ligaments, which attach from the ischial tuberosities and ischial spines bilaterally to the sacrum, respectively. Together, these ligaments contribute significantly to the stability of the pelvis.

The firm, soft tissue support of the pelvic floor consists of the muscles of the *pelvic diaphragm*, which is made up of the coccygeus muscles and levator ani muscles (pubococcygeus, puborectalis, and iliococcygeus).[1] The pubococcygeus muscle is further divided into its pubovaginalis, puboperinealis, and puboanalis portions, providing additional support to the urethra and anus, and helping to narrow the urogenital hiatus. The puborectalis muscle is a U-shaped muscular sling encircling the junction between the rectum and anus, which determines the resting anorectal angle and partially contributes to the fecal continence mechanism.[1] The lateral walls of the pelvis are formed by the piriformis muscle and obturator internus muscle. The piriformis muscle originates from the anterior and lateral surfaces of sacrum to fill, in part, the posterolateral pelvic walls. The obturator internus muscle originates on the pelvic surfaces of the ilium and ischium, and fills the remainder of the sidewalls of the pelvis. The *levator plate* is a clinical or conceptual term to describe the connection between the anus and the coccyx, formed by the medial insertions of the iliococcygeus muscle on the coccyx, known as the anococcygeal raphe.[1] As mentioned later, the levator plate is important in the discussion of theories of prolapse development, as it provides a ridge or shelf on which the rectum, upper vagina, and uterus rest.

Crucial to the discussion of pelvic floor support is the classification and distinction of ligamentous support and fascial layers within the pelvis (**Fig. 1**). Classically, fascia is designated as being either parietal or visceral.[1,2] Parietal fascia is thick, tough connective tissue that covers the medial surfaces of most skeletal or striated muscle in the pelvis; for example, the coccygeus and levator ani muscles. Importantly, parietal fascia may be freely dissected off of the underlying muscle. Special condensations of parietal fascia in the pelvis provide muscle attachments to the bony pelvis and anchoring points for visceral fascia.[1,2] Examples include the arcus tendineus levator ani (ATLA), arcus tendineus fascia pelvis (ATFP), and arcus tendineus fascia rectovaginalis (ATFR). In contrast, visceral fascia in the pelvis, also known as *endopelvic fascia*, provides subperitoneal perivascular connective tissue attachments from different pelvic visceral organs to the pelvic walls.[1] Under this classification, we find structures such as the uterosacral ligaments, cardinal ligaments, pubocervical/pubovesical fascia, and rectovaginal fascia. Herein lies controversy over the use of the term "fascia" in describing these visceral attachments, as it relates to the surgical repair of certain

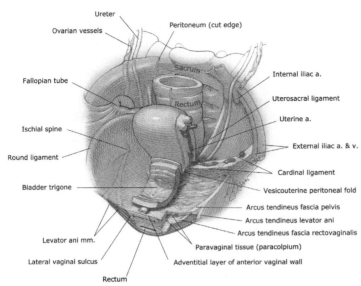

Fig. 1. Pelvic viscera and associated connective tissue support. Note distinction of the ATFP, ATLA, and ATFR, relative to the paracolpium. a, artery; mm, muscles; v, vein. (*From* Hoffman BL, Schorge JO, Schaffer JI, et al. Aspects of gynecologic surgery: anatomy. In: Calver L, editor. Williams gynecology. 2nd edition. New York: McGraw Hill; 2012. p. 931; with permission.)

vaginal wall defects.[2,3] In addition, the term "ligament" may be confusing, as the uterosacral and cardinal ligaments do not offer the same pelvic structural stability provided by the sacrospinous and sacrotuberous ligaments, for instance. These are important considerations, which are explored further throughout this review.

As described by DeLancey,[4] support of the bladder, vagina, uterus, and rectum in the pelvis is composed of a network of visceral connective tissue attachments that function as a continuous unit, but contain distinct areas that provide separate defined levels of support along the pelvic floor. For instance, the support of the uterus, or *parametria* (consisting of the broad, cardinal, and uterosacral ligaments), continues caudally, providing support of the vagina, or *paracolpium*. Our discussion of the concepts of pelvic floor support and prolapse in the separate vaginal compartments is therefore guided by the tissue interactions present at these different levels of vaginal support.

APICAL COMPARTMENT

In the apical compartment, the cervix and proximal third of the vagina are reinforced by what DeLancey[4] described as level I (suspension) support, which encompasses the upper paracolpium and functions to suspend the apex/upper third of the vagina to the walls of the pelvis. As noted previously, the paracolpium is a continuation of the parametria, which includes fibers of cardinal and uterosacral ligaments. The cardinal ligament, also known as the Mackenrodt or transverse cervical ligament, is made up of perivascular connective tissue and attaches the cervix and upper vagina to the posterolateral pelvic walls adjacent to the origin of the internal iliac artery, enveloping the vessels supplying the uterus and vagina.[5,6] The uterosacral ligament contains connective tissue, smooth muscle, and some autonomic pelvic nerve fibers.[7] The uterosacral ligaments originate at the posterior margin of the cervix and upper posterior vagina, extending from the S2 to the S4 vertebra of the sacrum.[8] Recently, in vivo dynamics of the cardinal and uterosacral ligament for apical support with and without Valsalva have been explored using 3-dimensional MRI.[9] These evolving imaging techniques continue to expand our knowledge of the strain and lengthening of these structures in living women, which in turn, may aid in determining the nature and direction of apical support loss.

According to the Integral Theory, the cardinal ligaments (laterally), pubocervical fascia (anteriorly), uterosacral ligaments (posterolateral), and the rectovaginal fascia (posteriorly) form the *pericervical ring*, providing support to the upper vagina.[10] These connective tissue relationships at the pericervical ring are demonstrated in **Fig. 2**. Failure of this cervical ring to support the bladder base leads to apical or middle compartment prolapse contributing to stress and urgency urinary symptoms. On physical examination, detachments of the anterior and posterior pericervical ring may be appreciated by assessing mobility and descent of the cervix. In addition, palpating the posterolateral aspects of the pericervical ring and visualizing bulging of the anterior or posterior fornices (indicating separation of the pubocervical or rectovaginal fascia, respectively) may aid in appreciating detachments at the pericervical ring.

An emerging concept in the discussion of apical compartment prolapse is that of cervical elongation/hypertrophy. Traditionally, pelvic organ prolapse is believed to be associated with some degree of cervical elongation, possibly due to the increasing pressures causing downward displacement and hypertrophy of the cervix. Berger and associates[11] used pelvic MRI to compare cervical lengths in women with and without prolapse, and found that women with prolapse have 36.4% longer cervices than women without prolapse. In addition, the amount of cervical elongation appeared to increase with greater degrees of uterine descent. However, clinical evaluation of cervical elongation remains difficult to assess and its significance is undetermined. The pelvic organ prolapse quantification (POP-Q) examination allows for precise and consistent evaluation of prolapse in distinct compartments, relative to fixed anatomic

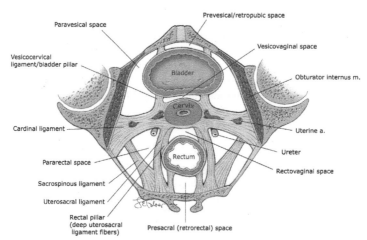

Fig. 2. Connective tissue and surgical spaces of the pelvis. Displayed are the connective tissues supports/ligaments contributing to the *pericervical ring*. The "pubocervical/pubovesical fascia" and "rectovaginal fascia" (not shown) are found in the vesicovaginal and rectovaginal spaces, respectively. a, artery. (*From* Hoffman BL, Schorge JO, Schaffer JI, et al. Aspects of gynecologic surgery: anatomy. In: Calver L, editor. Williams gynecology. 2nd edition. New York: McGraw Hill; 2012. p. 934; with permission.)

landmarks.[12] Ibeanu and colleagues[13] defined cervical elongation as a distance greater than 8 cm between points C and D. However, it may be inaccurate to assume that a large difference between points C and D implies presence of cervical elongation and may represent one of the limitations of the POP-Q system.[11] Recent studies have sought to examine the effectiveness of modifications to the POP-Q examination to help with preoperative diagnosis/assessment of cervical elongation.[14]

There are several important points regarding cervical elongation, support of the apical compartment, and impact on surgical decision-making. First, one may argue that significant cervical elongation in the presence of adequate apical support (as assessed by palpation of the uterosacral ligaments posteriorly) may only necessitate hysterectomy alone without a formal, restorative apical suspension. In addition, presence of significant cervical elongation combined with a large total vaginal length (10–12 cm) may impact a surgeon's approach when planning apical suspension via an abdominal sacrocolpopexy. In this setting, consideration must be given to performing either a total abdominal hysterectomy with upper vaginectomy or a supracervical hysterectomy with partial trachelectomy, so as to provide space for mesh placement between the apex and the fixation point on the sacrum. Last, procedures for prolapse with uterine preservation may actually require cervical amputation to improve outcomes.[15] This is especially important given emerging reports of significant cervical elongation developing after some uterine preservation procedures.[16,17]

In many ways, repair of prolapse in the apical compartment may be considered the "cornerstone" of a complete pelvic reconstruction.[18] This is in large part due to the importance of the integrity of the pericervical ring, where there is a convergence of the support mechanisms for the anterior, posterior, and apical compartments. Therefore, defects in apical support mechanisms are intimately related to defects in the anterior and posterior compartments. This may be demonstrated on physical examination, as simulated apical support during POP-Q examination reveals significant improvement of points Ba and Bp in 55% and 30% of women with stage II or greater prolapse.[19] Therefore, our discussion of the anterior and posterior compartments incorporates some of the same principles involved in apical support of the vagina.

ANTERIOR COMPARTMENT

The anterior compartment of the pelvic organ support system contains the urethra and bladder, adjacent to the anterior vaginal wall. It is separated from the posterior compartment by the vagina, uterus, and their associated supporting endopelvic fascia.[20] In addition to level I support at the pericervical ring, the anterior compartment receives level II (attachment) support via the lower paracolpium, offering suspension of the middle third of the vagina.[4] At the mid-vagina, the anterior wall has endopelvic fascial attachments to the ATFP, which provides a supportive layer beneath the bladder, also referred to as the pubocervical fascia. The ATFP is formed from the condensation of the fascia over the medial obturator internus and levator ani muscles, providing lateral attachment of the anterior vaginal wall to the pelvic sidewall. The distal third of the anterior compartment receives Level III (fusion) support via fusion of the pubocervical fascia to the perineal membrane, perineal body, and levator ani muscles.[4] As noted previously, the accuracy of using the term "pubocervical or pubovesical fascia" has been called into question given previous controversy over the existence of a separate layer of fascia between the bladder and vagina. However, more recent histologic studies of the anterior vaginal wall have not been able to validate a separate layer of fascia between the vagina and bladder.[3,21] Indeed, numerous cadaver studies have revealed that, histologically, the vesicovaginal space consisted of fibroadipose tissue containing nerves and vascular channels.[3,21,22] Therefore, the consensus now is that more appropriate terms to describe tissue being manipulated during repair of the anterior vaginal wall are "vaginal muscularis" or "fibromuscular wall."[1,2]

There have been evolving theories on the development of prolapse in the anterior compartment over time. White[23,24] described the idea of disruption and detachment of the lateral attachments to the ATFP, resulting in paravaginal defects. Later, Randall and Nichols[25] propagated the theory of distention and displacement: overdistention and attenuation of the anterior wall (due to vaginal delivery or atrophy) results in diminished rugal folds and wall thinning, followed by displacement of the wall inferiorly (due to detachment or elongation of the anterolateral attachments to the ATFP). Although the term cystocele was classically used to describe prolapse of the anterior compartment (because the bladder was commonly the structure behind the anterior vaginal wall), this has largely been replaced with the phrase "anterior wall defect." Later, further descriptions arose of distinct "breaks" in the "fascia" of the anterior vaginal wall, in the form of transverse (separation of the pubocervical fascia from the pericervical ring), midline (anteroposterior separation of fascia between bladder and vagina), and lateral (paravaginal) defects.[26] Despite these developments in our understanding of anterior compartment defects, repair of the anterior wall remains a challenge, with recurrence rates of 40% or higher with anterior colporrhaphy, prompting application of mesh augmentation procedures.[27–29]

Part of the challenge in approaching defects in the anterior compartment is difficulty in reliably identifying these defects based on physical examination. Clinical evaluation of anterior vaginal wall defects have been shown to have poor interexaminer and intraexaminer reliability, except in increasing stage prolapse.[30] The anterior compartment support is assessed by retracting the posterior vaginal wall with a split speculum. Defects in the endopelvic fascia support that manifest as anterior wall prolapse can be assessed by examining the vagina during Valsalva. The anterolateral vaginal sulci, the central/midline, and proximal/transverse portions of the anterior vaginal wall.[31] Giving temporary instrument support in these areas will often help distinguish the types of defects present. Other factors such as presence/absence of vaginal rugae also may suggest the location of certain anterior wall support defects.[32,33] Validated quantification techniques for assessing vaginal rugae have been described and may be useful for evaluating this parameter.[30] Finally, patient symptoms, such as incomplete bladder emptying and dysfunctional or obstructed voiding symptoms, may be indicators of prolapse severity.

More recently, theories have emerged regarding the associations between support of the anterior and apical compartments, which provide further insight into the complexity of anterior vaginal prolapse. Chen and associates[34] offered a biomechanical model using MRI imaging, demonstrating a "trap door" theory of combined prolapse in these compartments. According to this model, the magnitude of anterior vaginal wall prolapse is dependent on the degree of impairment sustained by the levator ani muscles and the cardinal/uterosacral ligament complex, in the presence of increasing intra-abdominal pressures. Diminished support via the levator ani muscles leads to downward rotation of the levator plate (trap door opens), widening of the urogenital hiatus, and worsening anterior vaginal wall prolapse and places the apical support on tension. Interestingly, 50% to 60% of anterior wall prolapse size is thought to be explained by apical descent, indicating that loss of apical support is a crucial factor in the development and/or progression of anterior wall prolapse.[35,36] In addition, MRI studies have shown that up to 77% of anterior wall prolapse can be attributed to apical descent and anterior vaginal wall length.[37] Studies comparing anterior colporrhaphy with and without mesh material, in the absence of a concomitant apical repair, have stimulated discussion regarding the association of defects in the anterior and apical compartments, and whether the repair of one necessitates the repair of the other.[38,39] Some have suggested that this association does not necessarily indicate or establish direct cause and effect.[39] It appears that the solution depends on the physical examination, because repair of the anterior wall alone may be sufficient if adequate support by the cardinal/uterosacral ligaments is found preoperatively. In contrast, concomitant apical repair may be required if there is significant loss of apical support in the presence of anterior wall prolapse.

Knowledge of these concepts is essential in assisting the surgeon with proper patient selection for specific approaches to the repair of prolapse in the anterior compartment. Special consideration should be given to whether or not a concomitant apical suspension is required to more effectively repair the anterior wall. Surgical options should remain individualized based on the patient's symptoms and physical examination.

POSTERIOR COMPARTMENT

The posterior compartment of the vagina contains the rectum and anus; it is separated from the anterior compartment by the vagina and uterus and their endopelvic attachments to the pelvic sidewalls. Level I support of the posterior compartment is shared with that of the anterior compartment (cardinal and uterosacral ligaments), which is reflected in the fact that proximally, the anterior and posterior vaginal walls abut, giving a flattened appearance on transverse cross section. In contrast, at the middle third of the vagina, the posterior compartment is supported by Level II support, via lateral endopelvic fascial attachments to the ATFR, preventing anterior expansion of the rectum.[20,40] These connections are analogous to the attachments of the anterior compartment to the ATFP, providing the characteristic H-shape of the mid-vagina on transverse cross section. The ATFR is a term proposed to describe the lateral attachments of "rectovaginal fascia" to the pelvic sidewall. It runs on the pelvic sidewall from the posterior fourchette to the ATFP, approximately midway between the ischial spine and pubic symphysis (**Fig. 3**).[40] The relationship of the ATFP and ATFR

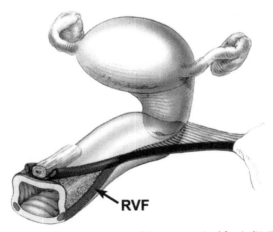

Fig. 3. ATFR. Shown as the lateral attachment of the rectovaginal fascia (RVF). (*From* Leffler KS, Thompson JR, Cundiff GW, et al. Attachment of the rectovaginal septum to the pelvic sidewall. Am J Obstet Gynecol 2001;185:43; with permission.)

is further demonstrated in **Fig. 4**. The distal third of the posterior compartment receives Level III (fusion) support via fusion of the "rectovaginal fascia" to the perineal membrane, perineal body, and levator ani muscles.[4]

Similar to the anterior compartment, the term "rectovaginal fascia," implying the presence of an actual "fascial" layer between the posterior vaginal wall and anterior rectum, has fallen out of favor. This layer is often also referred to as the rectovaginal septum or Denonvilliers fascia, which was described as a peritoneal remnant extending for 2 to 3 cm proximal to the perineal body and absent above the level of the posterior cul de sac.[2,41–43] However, histologic studies of the posterior compartment have been unable to consistently identify a separate fascial layer between the vagina and rectum.[44] These concepts are important surgically, because the idea of "fascial" layer may give the surgeon a false impression that there is more substantial or durable tissue than what is actually present.

Knowledge of these anatomic concepts is integral to understanding theories of prolapse development in the posterior compartment and identification of these defects. DeLancey[20] has provided intriguing concepts on the mechanics of support in the posterior compartment. Closure of the pelvic floor by the baseline contraction of the puborectalis muscle (which forms a sling around the rectum) draws the posterior vaginal wall against the anterior vaginal wall, allowing for balanced pressures on either wall upon Valsalva. Distally, there is no balancing of pressures and resistance of downward force upon Valsalva depends largely on the support of the perineal membrane/perineal body. With injury or impairment of the levator ani muscles, there are unbalanced pressures that generate a downward force on the posterior compartment, placing tension on the structures associated with level II support. Therefore, support of the posterior compartment is dependent on the dynamic interactions between the muscles and connective tissue attachments of the pelvic floor contributing to specific defects along its support system.

Classically, these defects were referred to as "rectoceles," which Richardson[43] described as isolated tears (midline, lateral, superior, or inferior) in the rectovaginal septum, visualized at the time of surgery. However, this term has largely been replaced by the term posterior wall prolapse or defect. These defects are analogous to those seen in the anterior compartment, corresponding to midline, paravaginal, and transverse defects that may be present in any combination. Repair of prolapse in the posterior compartment (posterior colporrhaphy) has been guided by the ability to recognize these defects preoperatively and intraoperatively.

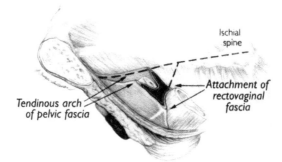

Fig. 4. The Y configuration formed by the junction of the ATFP and ATFR. (*From* Leffler KS, Thompson JR, Cundiff GW, et al. Attachment of the rectovaginal septum to the pelvic sidewall. Am J Obstet Gynecol 2001;185:42; with permission.)

On physical examination, the anterior wall is retracted with a split speculum, allowing for isolation of the posterior wall and assessment of rugal folds. Visualization of the position of the posterolateral sulci can help identify posterior paravaginal defects due to loss of lateral attachments to the ATFR. Importantly, in the upper third of the posterior compartment, peritoneum covers the surface of the rectovaginal fascia and in the middle third, the rectovaginal fascia abuts the posterior vaginal wall.[31] A rectovaginal examination may offer insight into the degree of impairment and detachments of the distal "rectovaginal fascia" to the perineal body, which may manifest as a perineal bulge or "low" posterior wall prolapse (also termed "perineocele" or "perineal rectocele"). In contrast, close inspection of a "high" posterior wall prolapse (also termed "enterocele") may show peristaltic movements of bowel under the vaginal epithelium, because breaks in the rectovaginal fascia facilitate descent of peritoneum directly against the vaginal wall with no intervening visceral fascia.[26,31] Therefore, high posterior wall defects are linked to loss of level I support to the pericervical ring and cardinal-uterosacral complex. Despite these observations, as with defects in the anterior compartment, the accuracy of the clinical evaluation of posterior compartment defects tends to be quite limited. Burrows and associates[45] discovered that preoperative examination of the posterior wall concurred with intraoperative descriptions of defects only 60% of the time.

Difficulties in identifying these specific defects clinically have prompted new investigations into the use of specific imaging techniques to assist in evaluation of posterior compartment defects, which may help direct the type of surgical approach chosen. Specifically, it may be difficult to correlate a patient's symptoms (ie, splinting for defecation) with what is seen on examination in the posterior compartment. Besides use of a pessary trial to check for alleviation of symptoms, in vivo imaging may sometimes provide useful information. Dynamic MR defecography has emerged as a method of objectively evaluating size of posterior wall prolapse, dysfunctional emptying, and identifying defects not easily seen on physical examination. Dynamic MRI has been shown to be useful for diagnosing an "enterocele" and differentiating it from a high rectocele, which may in turn affect the type of surgery needed for repair.[46] However, it remains imperative to correlate MRI findings with actual patient symptoms, which should ultimately guide surgical decision-making. Given the complexity of symptoms present with posterior compartment prolapse, oftentimes a multidisciplinary approach with gastroenterologists and colorectal and pelvic surgeons is needed to address functional or physiologic impairments, in addition to anatomic or mechanical impairments.

SUMMARY/DISCUSSION

The support network of the pelvic floor has been best described as being "continuous and interdependent."[4] Therefore, the evaluation and surgical approach to pelvic organ prolapse should include a comprehensive assessment of pelvic floor support. This requires expert-level knowledge of anatomy and a clear understanding of the mechanisms by which prolapse progresses. Ultimately, we must account for the global topography of the pelvic floor and correlate this with specific clinical symptoms. However, recognizing the separate concepts related to apical, anterior, and posterior prolapse might help surgeons to compartmentalize and focus their approach to diagnose and treat specific support defects.

ACKNOWLEDGMENTS

We acknowledge the artistic contributions of Lianne Krueger Sullivan and Lewis Calver, the medical illustrators for the reprinted figures displayed in this document.

REFERENCES

1. Corton MM. Aspects of gynecologic surgery. Chapter 38. Anatomy. In: Hoffman BL, Schorge JO, Schaffer JI, et al, editors. Williams gynecology. 2nd edition. New York: McGraw-Hill Medical; 2012. p. 917–47.
2. Corton MM. Anatomy of pelvic floor dysfunction. Obstet Gynecol Clin North Am 2009;36:401–19.
3. Weber AM, Walters MD. Anterior vaginal prolapse: review of anatomy and techniques of surgical repair. Obstet Gynecol 1997;89:311–8.
4. DeLancey JOL. Anatomic aspects of vaginal eversion after hysterectomy. Am J Obstet Gynecol 1992;166:117–28.
5. Range R, Woodburne R. The gross and microscopic anatomy of the transverse cervical ligament. Am J Obstet Gynecol 1964;90:460–7.
6. Iancu G, Doumouchtsis SK. A historical perspective and evolution of our knowledge on the cardinal ligament. Neurourol Urodyn 2014;33:380–6.
7. Campbell RM. The anatomy and histology of the sacrouterine ligaments. Am J Obstet Gynecol 1950;59:1–12.
8. Ramanah R, Berger MB, Parratte BM, et al. Anatomy and histology of apical support: a literature review concerning cardinal and uterosacral ligaments. Int Urogynecol J 2012;23:1483–94.
9. Luo J, Betschart C, Chen L, et al. Using stress MRI to analyze the 3D changes in apical ligament geometry from rest to maximal Valsalva: a pilot study. Int Urogynecol J 2014;25:197–203.
10. Petros PEP, Ulmsten UI. An integral theory of female urinary incontinence. Acta Obstet Gynecol Scand 1990;69:7–31.
11. Berger MB, Ramanah R, Guire KE, et al. Is cervical elongation associated with pelvic organ prolapse? Int Urogynecol J 2012;23:1095–103.
12. Bump RC, Mattiasson A, Bo K, et al. The standardization of terminology of female pelvic organ prolapse and pelvic floor dysfunction. Am J Obstet Gynecol 1996; 175:10–7.
13. Ibeanu OA, Chesson RR, Sandquist D, et al. Hypertrophic cervical elongation: clinical and histological correlations. Int Urogynecol J 2010;21: 995–1000.
14. Antovska SV. A new modification of the POPQ system–its effectiveness in the diagnosis of supravaginal elongation of the uterine cervix in cases with genital prolapse. Bratisl Lek Listy 2008;109:307–12.
15. Walters MD. Uterovaginal prolapse in a woman desiring uterine preservation. Int Urogynecol J Pelvic Floor Dysfunct 2008;19:1465–70.
16. Vierhout ME, Futterer JJ. Extreme cervical elongation after sacrohysteropexy. Int Urogynecol J 2013;24:1579–80.
17. Hyakutake MT, Cundiff GW, Geoffrion R. Cervical elongation following sacrospinous hysteopexy: a case series. Int Urogynecol J 2014;25:851–4.
18. Ross JW. Apical vault repair, the cornerstone or pelvic vault reconstruction. Int Urogynecol J Pelvic Floor Dysfunct 1997;8:146–52.
19. Lowder JL, Park AJ, Ellison R, et al. The role of apical vaginal support in the appearance of anterior and posterior vaginal prolapse. Obstet Gynecol 2008; 111:152–7.
20. DeLancey JOL. Structural anatomy of the posterior pelvic compartment as it relates to rectocele. Am J Obstet Gynecol 1999;180:815–23.
21. Ricci JV, Thom CH. The myth of a surgically useful fascia in vaginal plastic reconstructions. Q Rev Surg 1954;11:253–6.

22. Balgobin S, Hamid CA, Carrick KS, et al. Surgical anatomy of the anterior colpotomy/vesico-cervical space for vaginal hysterectomy. Abstract presented at 37th Annual Scientific Meeting of the Society of Gynecologic Surgeons. San Antonio, April 11–13, 2011.

23. White GR. Cystocele—a radical cure by suturing lateral sulci of the vagina to the white line of pelvic fascia. J Am Med Assoc 1909;21:1707–10.

24. White GR. An anatomical operation for the cure of cystocele. Am J Obstet Dis Women Child 1912;65:286–90.

25. Randall CL, Nichols DH. Surgical treatment of vaginal inversion. Obstet Gynecol 1971;38:327–32.

26. Richardson AC, Lyon JB, Williams NL. A new look at pelvic relaxation. Am J Obstet Gynecol 1976;126:568–73.

27. Sand PK, Koduri S, Lobel RW, et al. Prospective randomized trial of polyglactin 910 mesh to prevent recurrence of cystoceles and rectoceles. Am J Obstet Gynecol 2001;184:1357–64.

28. Weber AM, Walters MD, Piedmonte MR, et al. Anterior colporrhaphy: a randomized trial of three surgical techniques. Am J Obstet Gynecol 2001;185:1299–306.

29. Nguyen JN, Burchette RJ. Outcome after anterior vaginal prolapse repair. Obstet Gynecol 2008;111:891–8.

30. Whiteside JL, Barber MD, Paraiso MF, et al. Clinical evaluation of anterior vaginal wall support defects: interexaminer and intraexaminer reliability. Am J Obstet Gynecol 2004;191:100–4.

31. Cundiff GW. The clinical evaluation of pelvic organ prolapse. In: Bent AE, Cundiff GW, Swift SE, editors. Ostergard's urogynecology and pelvic floor dysfunction. 6th edition. Philadelphia: Lippincott Williams & Wilkins; 2008. p. 422–39.

32. Shull BL. Clinical evaluation of women with pelvic support defects. Clin Obstet Gynecol 1993;36:939–51.

33. Whiteside JL, Barber MD, Paraiso MF, et al. Vaginal rugae: measurement and significance. Climacteric 2005;8:71–5.

34. Chen L, Ashton-Miller JA, Hsu Y, et al. Interaction between apical supports and levator ani in anterior vaginal support: theoretical analysis. Obstet Gynecol 2006;108:324–32.

35. Summers A, Winkel LA, Hussain HK, et al. The relationship between anterior and apical compartment support. Am J Obstet Gynecol 2006;194:1438–43.

36. Rooney K, Kenton K, Mueller ER, et al. Advanced anterior vaginal wall prolapse is highly correlated with apical prolapse. Am J Obstet Gynecol 2006;195:1837–40.

37. Hsu Y, Chen L, Summers A, et al. Anterior vaginal wall length and degree of anterior compartment prolapse seen on dynamic MRI. Int Urogynecol J Pelvic Floor Dysfunct 2008;19:137–42.

38. Altman D, Vayrynen T, Engh ME, et al. Anterior colporrhaphy versus mesh for pelvic-organ prolapse. N Engl J Med 2011;364:1826–36.

39. DeLancey JOL. Surgery for cystocele III: do all cystoceles involve apical descent? Int Urogynecol J 2012;23:665–7.

40. Leffler KS, Thompson JR, Cundiff GW, et al. Attachment of the rectovaginal septum to the pelvic sidewall. Am J Obstet Gynecol 2001;185:41–3.

41. Denonvilliers C. Propositions et observations d'anatomie, de physiologie et de pathologie. Paris: impr et fonderie de Rignoux et Ce; 1837.

42. Kuhn RIP, Hollyock VE. Observations on the anatomy of the rectovaginal pouch and septum. Obstet Gynecol 1982;59:445–7.

43. Richardson AC. The rectovaginal septum revisited: its relationship to rectocele and its importance in rectocele repair. Clin Obstet Gynecol 1993;36:976–83.

44. Kleeman SD, Westermann C, Karram MM. Rectoceles and the anatomy of the posterior vaginal wall: revisited. Am J Obstet Gynecol 2005;193:2050–5.
45. Burrows LJ, Sewell C, Leffler KS, et al. The accuracy of clinical evaluation of posterior vaginal wall defects. Int Urogynecol J 2003;14:160–3.
46. Gupta S, Sharma JB, Hari S, et al. Study of dynamic magnetic resonance imaging in diagnosis of pelvic organ prolapse. Arch Gynecol Obstet 2012;286:953–8.

Anatomy of the Vulva and the Female Sexual Response

Jennifer Yeung, DO*, Rachel N. Pauls, MD

KEYWORDS

- Vulva • Clitoris • Anatomy • Female sexual pleasure • G-Spot • Arousal • Orgasm

KEY POINTS

- The vulva is a complicated anatomic structure intricately involved in the female sexual response cycle.
- The structures extend inferiorly from the pubic arch and include the mons pubis, labia majora, labia minora, vestibule, and clitoris.
- The clitoris is widely accepted as the most critical anatomic structure to female sexual arousal and orgasm.
- The female sexual response cycle is very complex, requiring emotional and mental stimulation in addition to end organ stimulation.
- With the increase of cosmetic procedures to alter the vulva, obstetricians and gynecologists are the experts in vulvar anatomy and function.

INTRODUCTION

The female vulva is an elaborate organ. Comprising several components, the vulvar structures act synergistically with mental well-being to enhance sexual response. Recent advancements in characterizing this intricate anatomy using both cadaveric dissection and MRI have furthered our knowledge. Nevertheless, the interplay of each part and their physiologic significance remain controversial.

Alongside these scientific advancements has been mounting interest regarding genital appearance. Complete pubic hair removal is widespread,[1] and labial photos and pornography are pervasive due to ease of Internet navigation.[2,3] Among Western cultures, studies have reported that nonprotruding and symmetric labia minora are perceived as normal for most men and women.[1,4] Resultant societal pressure to fit a particular physical ideal can harm female confidence and lower body image.

Disclosure Statement: None.
Female Pelvic Medicine and Reconstructive Surgery Fellowship Program, TriHealth Good Samaritan Hospital, 3219 Clifton Avenue, #100, Cincinnati, OH 45220, USA
* Corresponding author.
E-mail address: jennifer_yeung@trihealth.com

Obstet Gynecol Clin N Am 43 (2016) 27–44
http://dx.doi.org/10.1016/j.ogc.2015.10.011
0889-8545/16/$ – see front matter © 2016 Elsevier Inc. All rights reserved.

obgyn.theclinics.com

Mirroring this heightened scrutiny, cosmetic procedures to alter the vulva are on the rise. In fact, labiaplasty procedures in the United States increased 49% from 2013 to 2014; the second largest growth of a single surgical procedure over that period.[5] Furthermore, labiaplasty is only one of many procedures that are categorized as female genital cosmetic surgery, alongside vaginoplasty, perineoplasty, clitoral hood reduction, labial augmentation, and G-Spot amplification. Notably, more than half of US cosmetic surgeons now offer labiaplasty.[6]

Nevertheless, the providers with the most knowledge of the female anatomy and physiology remain the obstetricians/gynecologists. Surgical procedures may be harmful or unnecessary. Thus, the onus is on the obstetricians/gynecologists' field to remain the experts on counseling women about their bodies, sexual function, and appropriate options.[7]

VULVA

The structures that comprise the vulva extend inferiorly from the pubic arch and can be divided into nonerectile and erectile parts. Nonerectile parts include the mons pubis, labia majora, and vestibule of the vagina. Erectile parts include labia minora, clitoris, and clitoral bulbs (**Fig. 1**). The clitoris is of paramount importance and is discussed separately from the other structures.

Mons

The mons pubis is an inverted triangular area of fatty tissue covered with hair-bearing skin overlying the anterior aspect of the pubic bone. It extends from the glans clitoris inferiorly to the pubic hairline (the base of this triangle). The primary composition of the mons pubis is adipose tissue overlying fascia, which is a continuation of the Camper and Scarpa fascia from the anterior abdominal wall. The average length of the base is reported as 16 cm, and the average height of the triangle is 13 cm.[8,9]

Labia Majora

The labia majora (labium, singular) are prominent paired cutaneous lateral folds of hair-bearing skin and adipose tissue that extend inferiorly from the mons pubis and merge

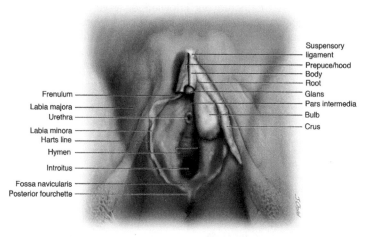

Fig. 1. Female vulva and clitoris. (*Adapted from* Pauls RN. Anatomy of the clitoris and the female sexual response. Clin Anat 2015;28(3):377; with permission.)

with neighboring skin to form a ridge overlying the perineal body, also known as the posterior fourchette.[10] Besides adipose tissue, they also contain the distal ends of the round ligaments, hair follicles, and a rich supply of sebaceous, apocrine, and eccrine sweat glands.[8,10] The lateral surfaces of the lips of the labia majora in the adult are covered with pigmented skin containing many glands and pubic hair, while the insides remain smooth, pink, and hairless.

Labia majora resemble the anterior abdominal wall in their underlying composition: Camper's fascia with a predominance of fat which is superficially located. The thicker Colles fascia forms the deeper layer and corresponds to the Scarpa fascia in the abdominal wall. The Colles fascia is inferiorly attached to the ischiopubic rami and posteriorly to the urogenital diaphragm, but lacks anterior attachments; this may be clinically significant, because hematomas and infections are is unable to extend to the thigh region, but may travel to the anterior abdominal wall.[8] The average length of the labia majora from the most superior aspect of the clitoral hood to the posterior fourchette ranges between 7 and 12 cm.[11]

Labia Minora

The labia minora are pigmented, hairless folds of skin, devoid of fat, but rich in nerve endings and sensory receptors. They are located medial to the labia majora immediately adjacent to the vestibule (see **Fig. 1**). Anteriorly, each separates into 2 folds that run over and under the glans of the clitoris. The superior folds unite in the midline to form the prepuce, or clitoral hood. The inferior folds insert into the underside of the clitoris to form the frenulum. The posterior aspects of both labia minora merge with the labia majora at the posterior fourchette. The Hart line demarcates the transition between the keratinized epithelium of the labia minora (embryologically deriving from the ectoderm) and the nonkeratinized epithelium of the vestibule of the vagina (embryologically deriving from the endoderm).[12]

The dermis of the labia minora is composed of thick connective tissue containing elastic fibers and small blood vessels. The arrangement of the blood vessels forms erectile tissue similar to the penile corpus spongiosum.[13] The labia minora are highly innervated along their entire edge, allowing detection of patterns at a very fine scale. A recent study has shown characteristic staining patterns of free nerve endings, Meissner corpuscles, and Pacinian corpuscles in the labia minora. Because of these innervation patterns, they may play a role in sexual sensation and arousal.[14,15] Furthermore, due to the termination of the labia minora at the clitoral hood, any traction or manipulation of the labia may stimulate the clitoris. This movement could contribute to sexual function and may be reduced following labial revision.[14] MRI studies of female organs during sexual arousal have demonstrated specific changes to the width of labia minora corresponding with their erectile behavior.[16]

There is a large variation in the dimensions of the labia minora; average length ranges from 2 to 10 cm, measured from the frenulum of the clitoris to the posterior fourchette, while the width varies from 0.7 to 5 cm, extending laterally from the hymen.[11] They may be asymmetrical or even duplicated on one or both sides.[17] In some African populations, labia minora have been stretched to 20 cm, while in Western societies today labiaplasty has been increasing in popularity.[17–19]

Vestibule

The vestibule of the vagina includes the area between the hymen and Hart line laterally, the frenulum of the clitoris anteriorly, and the posterior fourchette posteriorly. It contains the vaginal orifice, external urethral meatus, clitoral bulbs, the openings of the 2 greater vestibular (Bartholin) glands, and those of numerous, mucous, lesser vestibular glands.[20] The area between the frenulum of the clitoris and the external urethral meatus where the clitoral bulbs join together anteriorly is the female corpus spongiosum or pars intermedia.[21] The area between the hymen and posterior fourchette is the fossa navicularis (see **Fig. 1**). The external urethral meatus is located within the vestibule of the vagina superior to the vaginal opening. Two paraurethral Skene glands are located at the posterior-lateral aspect of the urethral meatus, line the urethra longitudinally, and aid in lubrication. The Bartholin glands open into the posterior-lateral aspect of the vestibule at approximately the 5 and 7 o'clock positions.[20]

The vestibule is an area of some significance in patients presenting with vulvar pain and dyspareunia. Although poorly understood, patients with these conditions often describe localized pain to the vestibule, which may occur either provoked or unprovoked. Patients with vulvar pain or vestibulodynia have been shown to have higher density of nerve endings in this tissue, which could be contributory. Moreover, the embryologic similarity with the lining of the urethra and bladder could help explain comorbidity with painful bladder and urethral syndromes.[22]

The hymen is a circumferential structure composed of non-hair-bearing skin. The internal surfaces of the hymen are normally in contact with each other and the vaginal orifice appears as a cleft between them.[13] It is variable in shape, sometimes appearing as a ring, at other times, a semilunar fold. Occasionally, it can even be absent. Once ruptured, the small skin elevations found in a circumferential pattern are referred to as hymeneal remnants.[23] Although there is no known function to the hymen, an unruptured hymen has cultural significance in many societies, because it is deemed proof of virginity.[24] Unfortunately, there is considerable variation in normal hymeneal appearance, and this tissue can be torn during tampon usage, speculum examination, and even athletic activity.[25–27] Despite these hymenal variations, hymenorrhaphy or hymenoplasty procedures for "revirgination" have been documented to re-create an intact hymen. Some describe cutting a flap off the back vaginal wall and bringing it across the vaginal opening to create "a band across the hymeneal ring," or even inserting a gelatin capsule containing fake blood that can burst on penetration.[28,29]

Innervation

The pudendal nerve is the main sensory and motor nerve of the perineum. It originates from the anterior rami of the second through fourth sacral nerve roots, runs under the piriformis, and exits the pelvis through the greater sciatic foramen. It then passes behind the ischial spine and re-enters the pelvis through the lesser sciatic foramen (**Fig. 2**). The pudendal nerve then runs in the Alcock canal (pudendal canal) in the obturator fascia and ventral to the sacrotuberous ligament.[30,31] As it enters the perineum, the pudendal nerve lies on the lateral wall of the ischiorectal fossa and divides into 3 branches: the inferior rectal, perineal, and dorsal nerve of the clitoris.[32]

The dorsal nerve of the clitoris lies on the perineal membrane along the ischiopubic ramus and on the anterolateral surface of the clitoris, one on each side, and supplies the clitoris.[33,34] The perineal nerve divides into several branches and supplies the external urethral sphincter, bulbocavernosus, ischiocavernosus, superficial transverse perineal muscles, and the skin of the medial portion of the labia majora, labia minora, and vestibule (**Fig. 3**). The inferior rectal nerve supplies the perianal skin and the external anal sphincter (see **Fig. 3**).

In addition to the branches of the pudendal nerve, innervation is also supplied by the cutaneous branch of the ilioinguinal nerve, the genital branch of genitofemoral nerve, and the perineal branch of the posterior femoral cutaneous nerve (see **Fig. 3**). Additional branches including the nerve to the levator ani and the accessory nerve to the

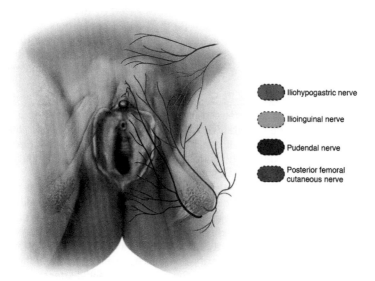

Fig. 2. Innervation to the clitoris and the vulva. (*From* Pauls RN. Anatomy of the clitoris and the female sexual response. Clin Anat 2015;28(3):381; with permission.)

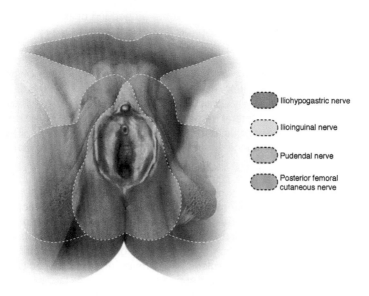

Fig. 3. Dermatomal distribution of the external female genitalia. (*From* Mazloomdoost DM, Pauls RN. A comprehensive review of the clitoris and its role in female sexual function. The Journal of Sexual Medicine 2015;3(4):248; with permission.)

perineal muscles and perianal skin have been reported by different investigators.[30] The bulbocavernosus reflex involves the S2 through S4 nerve roots. Gently tapping the clitoral prepuce stimulates the sensory afferent component of the dorsal nerve of the clitoris, which is transmitted to the motor efferent component of the inferior rectal nerve resulting in an anal wink.[35]

Vascular Supply

Arterial supply of the vulva is derived from the external and the internal pudendal arteries on each side. The vulva derives its vascular supply primarily from the internal pudendal artery, a branch of the internal iliac. The vein drains into the internal iliac vein. The vessels follow the course of the pudendal nerve and supply the superficial perineal muscles and external genitalia via different branches.[13]

The inferior rectal artery supplies the anal canal; the perineal artery supplies the superficial perineal muscles, posterior labial branch, artery to the bulb of the vestibule, dorsal and deep arteries of the clitoris; the urethral artery supplies the respective structures.[23] The superficial and deep external pudendal arteries are branches of the femoral artery; they distribute into the labia majora and anastomose with branches of the internal pudendal artery. There is a network of anastomosis between branches of these arteries throughout the female external genitalia. The external pudendal artery originates from the external iliac artery to supply the most superior aspect of the labia majora.[36]

CLITORIS

The complexity of the clitoris is often neglected despite being widely accepted as the most critical anatomic structure to female sexual arousal and orgasm.[33,37-39]

The clitoris actually consists of 6 main components: glans, suspensory ligament, body (corpora), root, paired crura, and vestibular bulbs (**Fig. 4**). Broadly, the clitoris has external and internal components that are embedded deep in the labia minora fat and vasculature and inferior to the pubic arch and symphysis. The external component of the clitoris consists of the glans, which is covered by the prepuce anteriorly and bordered by the frenulum posteriorly. The deeper, internal structures of the clitoris are the body, paired crura, and vestibular bulbs.[37,38,40,41] Both physiologically and anatomically, however, the clitoris has an intimate relationship with the distal urethra and vagina. The clitoris partially encircles the distal urethra, lies below the vestibular skin, and abuts the distal lateral vaginal walls. The term clitoral urethral complex and other variations have been used to describe this important area.[42,43] These structures share vasculature and innervation and move in unison during sexual activity.[39]

Glans, Prepuce, and Frenulum

The glans is the only external portion of the clitoris and thus has been anatomically described more often than any other part. It is a short cylindrical erectile organ in the superior portion of the vestibule. Its length varies from 1 to 2 cm and its diameter varies from 0.5 to 1 cm.[17,44] It is covered by the prepuce, which connects to the labia minora bilaterally by the frenulum, the demarcation of the labial skin, and the skin of the clitoris.[23] Microscopically, the glans is a fibrovascular cap of specialized genital vascular tissue that is distinct from and superficial to the erectile tissues of the corpora cavernosa of the clitoral body.[45] In fact, it contains the smallest segment of erectile tissue compared with other structures. Because of the absence of a tunica albuginea, hairless thin skin directly overlies the dense, vascular dermis of the glans.[42]

The somatic innervation of the glans is mediated by the dorsal nerve of the clitoris, a branch of the pudendal nerve (**Fig. 5**). It travels distally along the dorsal aspect of the

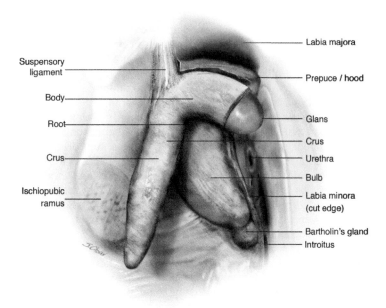

Suspensory ligament

Body

Root

Crus

Ischiopubic ramus

Labia majora

Prepuce / hood

Glans

Crus

Urethra

Bulb

Labia minora (cut edge)

Bartholin's gland

Introitus

Fig. 4. Components of the clitoral complex. (*From* Pauls RN. Anatomy of the clitoris and the female sexual response. Clin Anat 2015;28(3):378; with permission.)

clitoral body at the 11 o'clock and 1 o'clock positions before terminating in numerous corpuscular receptors in the subepithelial tissues.[33] Two distinct types of corpuscular receptors have been identified: genital end-bulb and Pacinian corpuscles.[38,46] Histologically, the glans has the largest number of small nerves when compared with other clitoral components, which supports its role in sensation.[42]

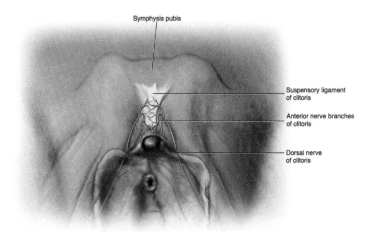

Symphysis pubis

Suspensory ligament of clitoris

Anterior nerve branches of clitoris

Dorsal nerve of clitoris

Fig. 5. Anatomic association of the suspensory ligaments and innervation of the clitoris. (*From* Pauls RN. Anatomy of the clitoris and the female sexual response. Clin Anat 2015;28(3):379; with permission.)

Body and Crura

The body of the clitoris is 1 to 2 cm wide and approximately 2 to 4 cm long. It initially extends cephalad and then folds back on itself in a boomerang-like shape before bifurcating at the pubic symphysis into the 2 crura in the "wishbone" configuration (see **Fig. 5**). Each crus is attached to the ischiopubic ramus laterally and below the skin of the labia minora.[38] The stems drape over the urethra and lay lateral to the vaginal walls. The crura are 5 to 9 cm long and narrower than the body.[40]

A dense connective tissue sheath, the tunica albuginea, surrounds the body of the clitoris, which is extremely vascular, comprising sinuses and smooth muscle trabeculae. The tunica albuginea has an incomplete midline septum dividing the clitoral body into 2 corpora. On the outer surface of the body lie branches of the dorsal nerves and vessels. In each erectile core of the corpora lie the deep clitoral arteries. Histology of the crura resembles that of the body in its type of erectile tissue, but it is not completely surrounded by a tunica and lacks the surrounding neurovascular structures and internal vasculature.[38] Microscopically, the body and crura contain the largest amount of erectile tissue but fewer nerves.[42]

Suspensory Ligament

In 1901, Poirier and Charpy[47] described the clitoral suspensory ligament as a "miniature representation" of the penile suspensory ligament. Several studies have now disputed this concept and have found it to be more substantial structure. The suspensory ligament of the clitoris is a thick, fibrofatty structure arising from the mons pubis in a fan shape (**Fig. 6**). The fibers extend from the deep fascia of the mons pubis and converge onto the body of the clitoris. The ligament extends down into the medial aspect of the labia majora in a sheetlike projection (see **Fig. 4**). The width of the superficial component is 7 to 8 cm and extends for 8 to 9 cm superficially and posteriorly to the clitoral glans. The deep component of the suspensory ligament extends from a narrow longitudinal origin on the pubic symphysis, converging on the superior and lateral aspects of the clitoral body, and then continuing deeply and posteriorly to attach on the bulbs. It has been found to be up to 1 cm in thickness.[34]

The suspensory ligament is hypothesized to support and restrict the movement of the body of the clitoris in a different manner than the ligaments of the male penis. As a result, the clitoris can rise upwards with arousal (erection), but cannot accomplish pendular motion and is unable to straighten.[23,34]

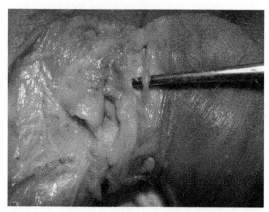

Fig. 6. Cadaveric dissection of the suspensory ligament. (*From* Pauls RN. Anatomy of the clitoris and the female sexual response. Clin Anat 2015;28(3):379; with permission.)

Root

The root of the clitoris is located below the skin of the vestibule and is the confluence of the clitoral erectile bodies, a zone highly responsive to direct stimulation and thus of great importance to female sexuality.[23]

Bulbs

The bulbs are contiguous structures with the glans and body of the clitoris. They are 2 erectile organs situated in the anterior region of the perineum. These paired structures fill the gap between the crura, body, and urethra. They are triangular in shape and 3 to 7 cm in length. The bulbs lay beneath the labia majora and against the distal vaginal wall. They engorge with arousal and thus may perform some lubricative function as well as stability to the vaginal walls.[40] This expansion may possibly bring the clitoral tissue closer to the vaginal lumen with arousal, which could aid in stimulation and sensation.[39]

Innervation

The clitoris is supplied by more than one set of nerves. The (somatic) pudendal nerve supplies the skin via the dorsal nerve of the clitoris while (visceral) fibers via the cavernous nerves supply arteries to erectile tissue.[23]

Clitoral innervation via bilateral terminations of the pudendal nerves arises at the pelvic sidewall.[33,38] The dorsal nerve of the clitoris travels inferior to the ischiopubic ramus to come close to the bundle from the contralateral side near midline. The paired nerves then enter the deep components of the suspensory ligament, which attaches to the clitoral body and pubic symphysis. At this point, the nerves are large, approximately 2 mm.[48] The nerves at the base of the clitoral body are suspended above the tunica and separated by approximately 5 to 10 mm into right and left trunks.[49] The 2 nerve trunks run at approximately the 11 o'clock and 1 o'clock positions in relation to the body within the suspensory ligament; no nerves are seen at the 12 o'clock position (**Fig. 7**). As the dorsal nerve of the clitoris travels distally toward the glans, it branches and fans out.[49] Nerve fibers then enter the glans beneath the corona.[48]

The cavernous neural anatomy is microscopic and much more difficult to define consistently. Studies have shown a network of nerves rather than discrete nerves.[40] The highest concentration of these small nerves has been found to be located within the mucosal surface of the glans, which supports the hypothesis that the glans is the area of highest sensation.[42]

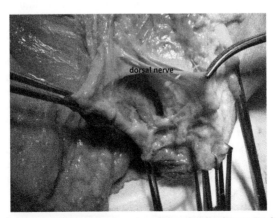

Fig. 7. Cadaveric dissection of the dorsal nerve of the clitoris. (*From* Pauls RN. Anatomy of the clitoris and the female sexual response. Clin Anat 2015;28(3):381; with permission.)

Vascular Supply

The blood supply of the clitoris arises from the pudendal vessels. The clitoris is supplied and drained from 4 directions: anteriolaterally and posterolaterally on both sides and is drained deep in the midline. The external pudendal supplies the prepuce, whereas the erectile components receive blood supply from the dorsal clitoral arteries, perineal arteries, and deep arteries. The deep dorsal vein in the clitoris drains the blood from the spaces in the corpora cavernosa into the vesical venous plexus.[23]

G-SPOT

Although descriptions of an erogenous zone in the anterior vaginal wall are described as far back as the first century AD in ancient Chinese and East Indian writings, it is only in more recent times the term "G-Spot" was used to describe a specific area that could be amplified or augmented to unlock female orgasm.[50] Because of the controversy surrounding the G-Spot, it is vitally important to understand its history.

In 1950, a German gynecologist named Ernst Grafenberg[51] published a report describing "the anterior wall of the vagina along the urethra" as "the seat of a distinct erotogenic zone." Although this early depiction did not garner high levels of attention, the concept was reintroduced in the 1980s via a case report of a woman who accomplished orgasm by digitally palpating a firm area along the course of the urethra. The investigators of that report concluded there to be an erogenous zone on the anterior vaginal wall and named it the "Grafenberg (G) spot."[52] Over the last few decades, this structure has received widespread attention yet little anatomic proof is documented, and scientists continue to debate its existence.[53,54]

Following this case report, Goldberg and colleagues[55] reported an area of the anterior vagina that swelled when stimulated and deemed this further confirmation of the spot. However, this area was documented in only 4 of 11 subjects in their study. Others have analyzed many different areas of the vagina and noted all can be sexually arousing, even to the level of orgasm.[56,57] Histologic research of vaginal mucosa dating back to the early 1950s has shown tissue rich in various discs, corpuscles, and nerve endings, but no specific G-Spot more richly innervated than other similar areas.[58] Later advanced techniques showed "no evidence for intraepithelial innervations," which would be expected if a sensitive G-Spot existed in that location.[59] Most recently, a group of scientists claimed the G-Spot as a neurovascular complex staining positive for SMA, CD31, and S100 that they described alongside the urethra.[60] Nevertheless, their conclusions seem unfounded, although nerve fibers in the vicinity of the vaginal wall are not unique and have been shown previously.[61]

Imaging studies have also been used to further understand the anterior vaginal wall and the potential G-Spot. Although the urethrovaginal space has been noted as thicker under ultrasound measurements in women with vaginal versus clitoral orgasms, it was unclear whether this was due to a G-Spot, or a consequence of stronger orgasmic contractions.[62] Newer imaging studies such as MRI have also been used to study the vagina, but the G-Spot has yet to be identified.[37,63–65]

The concept of female ejaculation/emission is also germane to this discussion because it has been used as evidence for the existence of the G-Spot. The only glandular structures in the G-Spot area are Skene glands, also known as the paraurethral glands.[66] These glands secrete various amounts of fluid during stimulation, which is biochemically similar to prostatic fluid.[67,68] Immunohistochemical staining also verifies that these glands correspond to prostate glands in prepubescent boys; as a result, some have proposed these glands be renamed the "female prostate."[69,70] Others argue that the G-Spot is actually this system of glands and ducts that play a role in sexual response and orgasm.[68,71] However, without confirmation of receptors for touch stimulation, such a relationship remains ill-defined.[72]

Further relevant to the phenomenon of the G-Spot is the question whether vaginal and clitoral orgasms are distinct entities. As noted earlier, the anatomy and location of the clitoris allow it to be stimulated from both external and internal manipulation.[73] Ultrasound examinations have shown that during perineal contraction, the anterior vaginal wall comes close to the clitoral root, and the root moves during penetration.[74] The position and size of the clitoris also appear to influence sexual response; a recent MRI study showed that women with normal orgasmic function had a larger clitoral glans and shorter distance from the vaginal lumen to the clitoris.[43] Most convincingly, however, are the reports of women born without a bladder or urethra, or following ritual genital mutilation, that describe sexual satisfaction (**Fig. 8**). These women likely retain the internal components of the clitoris, which in some situations may be reconstructed surgically.[75–78]

The importance of accurately describing the anatomy of the female genitalia is paramount in understanding female sexual gratification. The premise of the G-Spot, while unproven, is widely accepted to be real. Such misconceptions can lead to confusion regarding healthy sexual response, and pressure to achieve vaginal orgasm. In Western societies, the G-Spot has become a multimillion dollar industry, including books, movies, toys, and surgical intervention. Nevertheless, the American College of Obstetricians and Gynecologists advised against any cosmetic vaginal procedure without

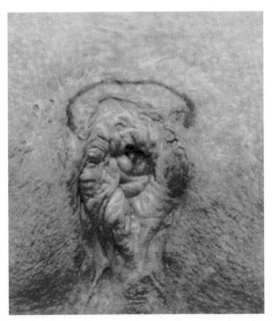

Fig. 8. 42-year-old woman born with congenital bladder exstrophy, who underwent cystectomy with bilateral ureterosigmoidostomy at the age of 2 years and distal neovaginoplasty at the age of 15 years. Note the absence of both urethra and visible clitoral glans. The photograph highlights her erotic areas marked in purple, a pelvic MRI was performed (image not shown) that confirmed these locations corresponded with clitoral tissue. (*Adapted from* Vaccaro CM, Herfel C, Karram MM, et al. Sexual function in a woman with congenital bladder exstrophy and multiple pelvic reconstructive surgeries: a case report. J Sex Med 2011;8(2):617–21; with permission.)

full disclosure of the potential risks and consequences, because such procedures are not routine surgical practice.[79]

FEMALE SEXUAL RESPONSE

Sexuality is basic to the human condition, and women rate sexuality as important to their quality of life.[80] Nevertheless, the female sexual response is complex, and there is likely no single model or cycle that applies to all women.

In the 1950s, Kinsey and colleagues[81] examined the sexual lives of women in the United States. Subsequently, Masters and Johnson[82] pioneered research efforts that expanded the scientific knowledge of the sexual response. They identified 4 physiologic stages: (1) excitement, (2) plateau, (3) orgasm, and (4) resolution. Later, a 3-phase model was proposed by Kaplan[83] consisting of (1) desire, (2) arousal, and (3) orgasm. Most recently, a circular female sexual response cycle has been proposed that integrates emotional intimacy, sexual stimuli, and relationship satisfaction.[84] There is no consensus; however, the fundamental components of desire, arousal, and orgasm are consistent.

Desire

Sexual desire, drive, or urge is one of the many reasons women initiate or agree to sexual intercourse.[85] Data from 125 women, aged 20 to 70, noted that all women identify triggers to sexual desire in the domains of emotional bonding, erotica, romance, and physical proximity.[86] Desire and arousal are difficult to distinguish as distinct entities, and desire does not always precede arousal. Desire can even be absent at the onset of sexual activity and then subsequently triggered during the actual sexual encounter. In fact, the baseline Study of Women Across the Nation reported most of 3262 multiethnic middle-aged women in North America were moderately or extremely satisfied with their physical sexual pleasure, yet never or infrequently sensed desire.[87]

Desire is thought to be triggered in the hypothalamus by activation of the dopamine system.[88–90] Research suggests that increased activity of the dopamine system occurs early in the sexual response and may propagate to and activate other areas of the brain, including the limbic system.[91]

Arousal

Sexual arousal in women results in increased genital blood flow, swelling of the labia and vaginal walls, release of lubricating secretions from the genital tract, and transudation from the subepithelial vasculature. The noradrenergic system is thought to be involved in the sexual arousal through the initiation of autonomic sensations of excitement resulting in increased heart rate and blood pressure (both systolic and diastolic).[92,93]

The sequence begins with stimulation of the sensory nerve fibers of the clitoris resulting in transmission through the sacral spinal cords. Vulvar blood flow increases from active neurogenic dilation of sinusoidal blood spaces in the corporal tissue of the clitoris, vestibular bulbs, and spongiosal tissue surrounding the urethra. Pelvic nerve stimulation results in clitoral smooth muscle relaxation and arterial smooth muscle dilation. With increasing arousal, parasympathetic stimulation causes dilation of the dorsal and deep arteries of the clitoris.[94]

Orgasm

Orgasm is a transient peak sensation of intense pleasure and can be described as a reflex. If sufficient arousal leads to orgasm, a reflex occurs that activates sympathetic fibers from T12 to L1 and waves of contraction of skeletal muscles may be mediated. Rhythmic contractions of the perineal, bulbocavernosus, and pubococcygeus muscles ensue, with sudden release of endogenous opioids, serotonin, prolactin, and oxytocin.[95,96] Although clitoral stimulation is not required to achieve orgasm, it has been shown to be an integral part of the orgasm reflex arc and may be the easiest and most common way to reach orgasm.[95,97] The 5 components of the reflex arc are (1) receptors of the clitoral complex and vulva, (2) somatic afferents of the pudendal nerves including the dorsal nerve of the clitoris and the perineal branches, (3) spinal cord nerve roots S2-S4, (4) visceral parasympathetic efferent fibers, and (5) the end organ of erectile tissue: clitoral complex, subbulbar, and urethral glands.[23]

There is also evidence that orgasm not only is a spinal reflex but also may involve the cerebral cortex as well. The earliest studies used electroencephalogram to show activity changes in this area.[98,99] Reports have been published on women with complete spinal cord injury who claimed they could perceive genital sensations, including orgasm.[100,101] A functional MRI study then found areas of both increased and decreased activity related to orgasm in both men and women.[102,103] Various studies since then have found conflicting information, but many of these studies used different imaging techniques, different stimulation methods, and different genital organ stimulation.

Resolution

Resolution has been associated with increased brain serotonergic activity and decreased dopamine release.[90] Resolution results in sympathetic arterial constriction and venous decongestion. The musculature then returns to basal tone.

SUMMARY

As physicians caring for female patients, we are obligated to understand, to the best of our ability, the anatomy and function of the vulva so that we may provide counsel on both appearance and purpose. Although the surgical alteration of the vulva is not a new practice, it is now more widely available than ever before. The female sexual response cycle has been shown to be more complex than just a 3-step model; it requires not just the stimulation of the end organ but also stimulation of the brain. Although physical appearance and body image are intricately linked to sexual confidence, the mind's understanding of the functionality of our body is stronger than any physical alteration will ever be. Through continued dedication to research of the female anatomy and education of our patients, women will be empowered to make the right decisions.

REFERENCES

1. Yurteri-Kaplan LA, Antosh DD, Sokol AI, et al. Interest in cosmetic vulvar surgery and perception of vulvar appearance. Am J Obstet Gynecol 2012;207(5): 428.e1–7.
2. Koning M, Zeijlmans IA, Bouman TK, et al. Female attitudes regarding labia minora appearance and reduction with consideration of media influence. Aesthet Surg J 2009;29(1):65–71.
3. McGregor JC. Labial surgery–a new phenomenon? J Plast Reconstr Aesthet Surg 2009;62(3):289.
4. Mazloomdoost D, Crisp CC, Westermann LB, et al. Survey of male perceptions regarding the vulva. Am J Obstet Gynecol 2015;213(5):731.e1–9.

5. Cosmetic Surgery National Data Bank Statistics. 2014. Available at: http://www. surgery.org/sites/default/files/2014-Stats.pdf.

6. Mirzabeigi MN, Moore JH Jr, Mericli AF, et al. Current trends in vaginal labioplasty: a survey of plastic surgeons. Ann Plast Surg 2012;68(2):125–34.

7. Pauls RN. We are the correct physicians to treat women requesting labiaplasty. Am J Obstet Gynecol 2014;211(3):218–218.e1.

8. Yavagal S, de Farias TF, Medina CA, et al. Normal vulvovaginal, perineal, and pelvic anatomy with reconstructive considerations. Semin Plast Surg 2011;25(2):121–9.

9. Seitz IA, Wu C, Retzlaff K, et al. Measurements and aesthetics of the mons pubis in normal weight females. Plast Reconstr Surg 2010;126(1):46e–8e.

10. Healy JC. Female reproductive system. In: Standring S, editor. Gray's anatomy. Edinburgh: Churchill Livingstone/Elsevier; 2008. p. 1279–304.

11. Lloyd J, Crouch NS, Minto CL, et al. Female genital appearance: "normality" unfolds. BJOG 2005;112(5):643–6.

12. Robboy SJ, Ross JS, Prat J, et al. Urogenital sinus origin of mucinous and ciliated cysts of the vulva. Obstet Gynecol 1978;51(3):347–51.

13. Williams PL, Bannister LH, Berry MM, et al. Gray's anatomy. New York: Churchill Livingstone; 1995.

14. Schober J, Aardsma N, Mayoglou L, et al. Terminal innervation of female genitalia, cutaneous sensory receptors of the epithelium of the labia minora. Clin Anat 2015;28(3):392–8.

15. Schober J, Cooney T, Pfaff D, et al. Innervation of the labia minora of prepubertal girls. J Pediatr Adolesc Gynecol 2010;23(6):352–7.

16. Suh DD, Yang CC, Cao Y, et al. MRI of female genital and pelvic organs during sexual arousal. J Psychosom Obstet Gynaecol 2004;25(2):153–62.

17. Dickinson R. Atlas of human sex anatomy. 2nd edition. Baltimore (MD): Williams & Williams; 1949.

18. Rouzier R, Louis-Sylvestre C, Paniel BJ, et al. Hypertrophy of labia minora: experience with 163 reductions. Am J Obstet Gynecol 2000;182(1 Pt 1):35–40.

19. Ellsworth WA, Rizvi M, Smith B, et al. Labia minora reduction: guidelines for procedure choice. Plast Reconstr Surg 2010;125(5):216e–7e.

20. Moore KL, Dalley AF. Clinically oriented anatomy. 4th edition. Baltimore (MD): Lippincott Williams & Wilkins; 1999.

21. van Turnhout AA, Hage JJ, van Diest PJ. The female corpus spongiosum revisited. Acta Obstet Gynecol Scand 1995;74(10):767–71.

22. Cervigni M, Natale F. Gynecological disorders in bladder pain syndrome/interstitial cystitis patients. Int J Urol 2014;21(Suppl 1):85–8.

23. O'Connell HE, Eizenberg N, Rahman M, et al. The anatomy of the distal vagina: towards unity. J Sex Med 2008;5(8):1883–91.

24. Hobday AJ, Haury L, Dayton PK. Function of the human hymen. Med Hypotheses 1997;49(2):171–3.

25. Goodyear-Smith FA, Laidlaw TM. What is an 'intact' hymen? A critique of the literature. Med Sci Law 1998;38(4):289–300.

26. Goodyear-Smith FA, Laidlaw TM. Can tampon use cause hymen changes in girls who have not had sexual intercourse? A review of the literature. Forensic Sci Int 1998;94(1–2):147–53.

27. Adams JA, Botash AS, Kellogg N. Differences in hymenal morphology between adolescent girls with and without a history of consensual sexual intercourse. Arch Pediatr Adolesc Med 2004;158(3):280–5.

28. Renganathan AC, Cartright R, Cardozo I. Gynecological cosmetic surgery. Expert Rev Obstet Gynecol 2009;4(2):101–4.

29. Cook RJ, Dickens BM. Hymen reconstruction: ethical and legal issues. Int J Gynaecol Obstet 2009;107(3):266–9.
30. Mahakkanukrauh P, Surin P, Vaidhayakarn P. Anatomical study of the pudendal nerve adjacent to the sacrospinous ligament. Clin Anat 2005;18(3):200–5.
31. Shafik A, el-Sherif M, Youssef A, et al. Surgical anatomy of the pudendal nerve and its clinical implications. Clin Anat 1995;8(2):110–5.
32. Schraffordt SE, Tjandra JJ, Eizenberg N, et al. Anatomy of the pudendal nerve and its terminal branches: a cadaver study. ANZ J Surg 2004;74(1–2):23–6.
33. Baskin LS, Erol A, Li YW, et al. Anatomical studies of the human clitoris. J Urol 1999;162(3 Pt 2):1015–20.
34. Rees MA, O'Connell HE, Plenter RJ, et al. The suspensory ligament of the clitoris: connective tissue supports of the erectile tissues of the female urogenital region. Clin Anat 2000;13(6):397–403.
35. Yucel S, De Souza A Jr, Baskin LS. Neuroanatomy of the human female lower urogenital tract. J Urol 2004;172(1):191–5.
36. Jin B, Hasi W, Yang C, et al. A microdissection study of perforating vessels in the perineum: implication in designing perforator flaps. Ann Plast Surg 2009;63(6): 665–9.
37. Suh DD, Yang CC, Cao Y, et al. Magnetic resonance imaging anatomy of the female genitalia in premenopausal and postmenopausal women. J Urol 2003; 170(1):138–44.
38. O'Connell HE, Sanjeevan KV, Hutson JM. Anatomy of the clitoris. J Urol 2005; 174(4 Pt 1):1189–95.
39. Jannini EA, Buisson O, Rubio-Casillas A. Beyond the G-spot: clitourethrovaginal complex anatomy in female orgasm. Nat Rev Urol 2014;11(9):531–8.
40. O'Connell HE, Hutson JM, Anderson CR, et al. Anatomical relationship between urethra and clitoris. J Urol 1998;159(6):1892–7.
41. Puppo V. Anatomy and physiology of the clitoris, vestibular bulbs, and labia minora with a review of the female orgasm and the prevention of female sexual dysfunction. Clin Anat 2013;26(1):134–52.
42. Oakley SH, Mutema GK, Crisp CC, et al. Innervation and histology of the clitoral-urethral complex: a cross-sectional cadaver study. J Sex Med 2013;10(9): 2211–8.
43. Oakley SH, Vaccaro CM, Crisp CC, et al. Clitoral size and location in relation to sexual function using pelvic MRI. J Sex Med 2014;11(4):1013–22.
44. Verkauf BS, Von Thron J, O'Brien WF. Clitoral size in normal women. Obstet Gynecol 1992;80(1):41–4.
45. Shih C, Cold CJ, Yang CC. Cutaneous corpuscular receptors of the human glans clitoris: descriptive characteristics and comparison with the glans penis. J Sex Med 2013;10(7):1783–9.
46. Halata Z, Munger BL. The neuroanatomical basis for the protopathic sensibility of the human glans penis. Brain Res 1986;371(2):205–30.
47. Poirier P, Charpy A. Traité d'anatomie humaine. In: Masson, editor. Vol 5. Paris. p 580.
48. Ginger VA, Cold CJ, Yang CC. Surgical anatomy of the dorsal nerve of the clitoris. Neurourol Urodyn 2011;30(3):412–6.
49. Vaze A, Goldman H, Jones JS, et al. Determining the course of the dorsal nerve of the clitoris. Urology 2008;72(5):1040–3.
50. Korda JB, Goldstein SW, Sommer F. The history of female ejaculation. J Sex Med 2010;7(5):1965–75.
51. Grafenberg E. The role of urethra in female orgasm. Int J Sexology 1950;3: 145–8.

52. Addiego FB, Belzer EG Jr, Comolli J, et al. Female ejaculation: a case study. J Sex Res 1981;17:13–21.
53. Pauls RN. Anatomy of the clitoris and the female sexual response. Clin Anat 2015;28(3):376–84.
54. Hines TM. The G-spot: a modern gynecologic myth. Am J Obstet Gynecol 2001; 185(2):359–62.
55. Goldberg DC, Whipple B, Fishkin RE, et al. The Grafenberg spot and female ejaculation: a review of initial hypotheses. J Sex Marital Ther 1983;9(1):27–37.
56. Alzate H, Londono ML. Vaginal erotic sensitivity. J Sex Marital Ther 1984;10(1): 49–56.
57. Alzate H. Vaginal eroticism: a replication study. Arch Sex Behav 1985;14(6): 529–37.
58. Krantz KE. Innervation of the human vulva and vagina; a microscopic study. Obstet Gynecol 1958;12(4):382–96.
59. Hilliges M, Falconer C, Ekman-Ordeberg G, et al. Innervation of the human vaginal mucosa as revealed by PGP 9.5 immunohistochemistry. Acta Anat (Basel) 1995;153(2):119–26.
60. Ostrzenski A, Krajewski P, Ganjei-Azar P, et al. Verification of the anatomy and newly discovered histology of the G-spot complex. BJOG 2014;121(11):1333–9.
61. Pauls R, Mutema G, Segal J, et al. A prospective study examining the anatomic distribution of nerve density in the human vagina. J Sex Med 2006;3(6):979–87.
62. Gravina GL, Brandetti F, Martini P, et al. Measurement of the thickness of the ure-throvaginal space in women with or without vaginal orgasm. J Sex Med 2008; 5(3):610–8.
63. Gutman RE, Pannu HK, Cundiff GW, et al. Anatomic relationship between the vaginal apex and the bony architecture of the pelvis: a magnetic resonance imaging evaluation. Am J Obstet Gynecol 2005;192(5):1544–8.
64. Schultz WW, van Andel P, Sabelis I, et al. Magnetic resonance imaging of male and female genitals during coitus and female sexual arousal. BMJ 1999; 319(7225):1596–600.
65. Yang CC, Cold CJ, Yilmaz U, et al. Sexually responsive vascular tissue of the vulva. BJU Int 2006;97(4):766–72.
66. Baggish MS, Karram M. Atlas of pelvic anatomy and gynecologic surgery. 3rd edition. St Louis (MO): Elsevier Saunders; 2011.
67. Shafik A, Shafik IA, El Sibai O, et al. An electrophysiologic study of female ejac-ulation. J Sex Marital Ther 2009;35(5):337–46.
68. Wimpissinger F, Stifter K, Grin W, et al. The female prostate revisited: perineal ultrasound and biochemical studies of female ejaculate. J Sex Med 2007;4(5): 1388–93 [discussion: 1393].
69. Wernert N, Albrech M, Sesterhenn I, et al. The 'female prostate': location, morphology, immunohistochemical characteristics and significance. Eur Urol 1992;22(1):64–9.
70. Puppo V, Puppo G. Anatomy of sex: revision of the new anatomical terms used for the clitoris and the female orgasm by sexologists. Clin Anat 2015;28(3): 293–304.
71. Darling CA, Davidson JK Sr, Conway-Welch C. Female ejaculation: perceived origins, the Grafenberg spot/area, and sexual responsiveness. Arch Sex Behav 1990;19(1):29–47.
72. Davidson JK Sr, Darling CA, Conway-Welch C. The role of the Grafenberg Spot and female ejaculation in the female orgasmic response: an empirical analysis. J Sex Marital Ther 1989;15(2):102–20.

73. Komisaruk BR, Wise N, Frangos E, et al. Women's clitoris, vagina, and cervix mapped on the sensory cortex: fMRI evidence. J Sex Med 2011;8(10):2822–30.
74. Foldes P, Buisson O. The clitoral complex: a dynamic sonographic study. J Sex Med 2009;6(5):1223–31.
75. Lightfoot-Klein H, Shaw E. Special needs of ritually circumcised women patients. J Obstet Gynecol Neonatal Nurs 1991;20(2):102–7.
76. Okonofu FE, Larsen U, Oronsaye F, et al. The association between female genital cutting and correlates of sexual and gynaecological morbidity in Edo State, Nigeria. BJOG 2002;109(10):1089–96.
77. Catania L, Abdulcadir O, Puppo V, et al. Pleasure and orgasm in women with female genital mutilation/cutting (FGM/C). J Sex Med 2007;4(6):1666–78.
78. Vaccaro CM, Herfel C, Karram MM, et al. Sexual function in a woman with congenital bladder exstrophy and multiple pelvic reconstructive surgeries: a case report. J Sex Med 2011;8(2):617–21.
79. Committee on Gynecologic Practice, American College of Obstetricians and Gynecologists. ACOG Committee Opinion No. 378: vaginal "rejuvenation" and cosmetic vaginal procedures. Obstet Gynecol 2007;110(3):737–8.
80. Naeinian MR, Shaeiri MR, Hosseini FS. General health and quality of life in patients with sexual dysfunctions. Urol J 2011;8(2):127–31.
81. Kinsey AC, Pomeroy WB, Martin CE, et al. Sexual behaviour in the human female. Philadelphia: W.B. Saunders Company; 1953.
82. Masters WH, Johnson VE. Human sexual response. Boston: Little Brown; 1966.
83. Kaplan H. Disorders of sexual desire. New York: Simon & Schuster; 1979.
84. Basson R, Leiblum S, Brotto L, et al. Definitions of women's sexual dysfunction reconsidered: advocating expansion and revision. J Psychosom Obstet Gynaecol 2003;24(4):221–9.
85. Stephenson KR, Ahrold TK, Meston CM. The association between sexual motives and sexual satisfaction: gender differences and categorical comparisons. Arch Sex Behav 2011;40(3):607–18.
86. McCall K, Meston C. Differences between pre- and postmenopausal women in cues for sexual desire. J Sex Med 2007;4(2):364–71.
87. Cain VS, Johannes CB, Avis NE, et al. Sexual functioning and practices in a multi-ethnic study of midlife women: baseline results from SWAN. J Sex Res 2003;40(3):266–76.
88. Gizewski ER, Krause E, Karama S, et al. There are differences in cerebral activation between females in distinct menstrual phases during viewing of erotic stimuli: a fMRI study. Exp Brain Res 2006;174(1):101–8.
89. Bartels A, Zeki S. The neural correlates of maternal and romantic love. Neuroimage 2004;21(3):1155–66.
90. Lorrain DS, Riolo JV, Matuszewich L, et al. Lateral hypothalamic serotonin inhibits nucleus accumbens dopamine: implications for sexual satiety. J Neurosci 1999; 19(17):7648–52.
91. Lorrain DS, Arnold GM, Vezina P. Mesoaccumbens dopamine and the self-administration of amphetamine. Ann N Y Acad Sci 1999;877:820–2.
92. Jeong GW, Park K, Youn G, et al. Assessment of cerebrocortical regions associated with sexual arousal in premenopausal and menopausal women by using BOLD-based functional MRI. J Sex Med 2005;2(5):645–51.
93. Exton MS, Bindert A, Krüger T, et al. Cardiovascular and endocrine alterations after masturbation-induced orgasm in women. Psychosom Med 1999;61(3):280–9.
94. Davis SR, Guay AT, Shifren JL, et al. Endocrine aspects of female sexual dysfunction. J Sex Med 2004;1(1):82–6.

95. Meston CM, Levin RJ, Sipski ML, et al. Women's orgasm. Annu Rev Sex Res 2004;15:173–257.

96. Shifren JL, Schiff I. Role of hormone therapy in the management of menopause. Obstet Gynecol 2010;115(4):839–55.

97. Singer I, Singer J. Periodicity of sexual desire in relation to time of ovulation in women. J Biosoc Sci 1972;4(4):471–81.

98. Cohen HD, Rosen RC, Goldstein L. Electroencephalographic laterality changes during human sexual orgasm. Arch Sex Behav 1976;5(3):189–99.

99. Graber B, Rohrbaugh JW, Newlin DB, et al. EEG during masturbation and ejaculation. Arch Sex Behav 1985;14(6):491–503.

100. Cole TM. Spinal cord injury patients and sexual dysfunction. Arch Phys Med Rehabil 1975;56(1):11–2.

101. Whipple B, Josimovich JB, Komisaruk BR. Sensory thresholds during the antepartum, intrapartum and postpartum periods. Int J Nurs Stud 1990;27(3): 213–21.

102. Georgiadis JR, Reinders AA, Paans AM, et al. Men versus women on sexual brain function: prominent differences during tactile genital stimulation, but not during orgasm. Hum Brain Mapp 2009;30(10):3089–101.

103. Georgiadis JR, Farrell MJ, Boessen R, et al. Dynamic subcortical blood flow during male sexual activity with ecological validity: a perfusion fMRI study. Neuroimage 2010;50(1):208–16.

Stress Urinary Incontinence
Comparative Efficacy Trials

Erin Seifert Lavelle, MD[a],*, Halina M. Zyczynski, MD[b]

KEYWORDS

- Stress urinary incontinence (SUI) • Treatment • Comparative efficacy • Review

KEY POINTS

- Weight loss of 5% to 10% of body weight results in more than 50% reduction in weekly stress urinary incontinence episodes.
- Approximately half of women with stress urinary incontinence experience symptom improvement from pelvic floor muscle therapy, compared with less than 10% with expectant management, and 91% after midurethral sling.
- Up to half of women who receive pelvic floor muscle therapy as initial treatment of moderate to severe stress urinary incontinence subsequently pursue surgical management. Surgery offered as first-line intervention is more likely to result in continence and treatment satisfaction in a shorter interval.
- Both retropubic and transobturator approaches to midurethral sling are highly successful procedures for stress urinary incontinence, with high long-term patient satisfaction. Adverse event profiles differ between approaches.
- Patients with contraindications or aversion to surgical mesh can be reassured that a Burch colposuspension or fascial pubovaginal sling result in similar continence rates and perioperative complications compared with midurethral slings.

INTRODUCTION

Almost 16% of community dwelling women in the United States report symptoms of urinary incontinence.[1] Most of these women report symptoms of stress urinary incontinence (SUI), or involuntary urine loss associated with coughing, sneezing, or other physical activity, without a preceding detrusor contraction.[2–4] Some women

Disclosure: The authors have nothing to disclose.
[a] Female Pelvic Medicine and Reconstructive Surgery, Department of Obstetrics, Gynecology and Reproductive Sciences, University of Pittsburgh School of Medicine, 300 Halket Street, Pittsburgh, PA 15213, USA; [b] Division of Urogynecology and Pelvic Reconstructive Surgery, Department of Obstetrics, Gynecology and Reproductive Sciences, University of Pittsburgh School of Medicine, 300 Halket Street, Pittsburgh, PA 15213, USA
* Corresponding author.
E-mail address: seifertee@upmc.edu

experience only stress-type incontinence, whereas many others report additional leakage symptoms such as urgency urinary incontinence (UUI), or leakage following a sudden and urgent need to void secondary to detrusor spasm. The combination of incontinence mechanisms is referred to as mixed urinary incontinence (MUI). SUI results in significant personal and financial burden for symptomatic women. Three-quarters of women who experience SUI report significant bother from their symptoms, and an estimated 13.6% of American women elect to undergo surgical treatment of SUI.[5]

Management strategies to reduce the burden of SUI include behavioral changes, weight reduction, pelvic floor muscle therapy (PFMT), and various surgical interventions. This article reviews the highest-quality clinical trials comparing contemporary treatment options for women with SUI. When available, results from large multicenter randomized controlled trials (RCTs) are highlighted. In their absence, results from smaller and single-site RCTs are reported, acknowledging their limitations. Clinicians and patients can use this compendium of the highest-quality studies to inform their treatment selection. For each trial, the population characteristics, number of participants, intervention, primary outcome, and notable secondary outcomes are presented. Where systematic reviews or meta-analyses are available, their findings are included as well.

NONSURGICAL MANAGEMENT FOR STRESS URINARY INCONTINENCE

Nonsurgical management strategies targeting SUI offer patients the potential for symptom improvement while avoiding the risk of surgical morbidity, such as perioperative complications, postoperative voiding dysfunction, or mesh exposure. The interventions in this class use behavior or lifestyle modifications such as bladder training, fluid management, and weight loss. Physical therapy targeting optimization of pelvic floor function, often referred to as PFMT, and incontinence pessaries are adjuvants to behavioral modifications. Outcomes of these strategies, used individually or in combination as first-line therapy, were investigated in several randomized trials. Fluid management, a keystone of behavior intervention for bladder symptoms, entails moderating total fluid intake and specifically bladder irritants such as caffeine and alcohol. Fluid management has not been addressed in a clinical trial for SUI treatment. Remaining treatments are addressed later.

Weight Loss

Overweight and obese women who lose 5% to 10% of their body weight can expect significant improvement in SUI.

Obesity is a risk factor for incontinence and imparts a 3-fold to 4-fold risk for SUI.[6,7] Sustained weight reduction among obese and morbidly obese women has shown substantial improvement in their incontinence symptoms in 2 large trials.

The Program to Reduce Incontinence by Diet and Exercise (PRIDE) study randomized 338 women to an intensive 6-month behavioral weight loss program versus a control treatment of 4 educational sessions on weight loss and healthy diet.[8] Both groups received an instruction booklet describing pelvic floor strengthening, incontinence suppression techniques, and bladder diaries. The primary outcome was weekly episodes of SUI reported by bladder diary at 6 months. Women in the weight loss group lost an average of 8% of their body weight, compared with 1.6% in the control group. The mean loss of 8% body weight was associated with a 58% reduction in weekly SUI episodes compared with 33% for controls (P = .01) at 6 months. Women in either group who maintained a 5% to 10% weight loss at 18 months were more than twice as likely as those who gained or maintained their weight to report a 70% reduction in symptoms, which was the investigators' a priori definition of clinically significant improvement in incontinence.[9] Women in the control arm perceived a 53% decrease in frequency of incontinence episodes when measured by Likert scale following the control interventions alone, despite minimal mean weight loss.

A beneficial effect of weight reduction on stress incontinence was also shown by the Action for Health in Diabetes (AHEAD) study of 2739 women with type 2 diabetes and a 13% prevalence rate of SUI.[10] Women were randomized to an intensive lifestyle modification weight loss program versus diabetes support and education, resulting in average weight loss of 7.7 kg compared with 0.7 kg respectively ($P = .01$). At 1 year, women in the study group were less likely to report new SUI symptoms (3.8% vs 6.2%, $P = .01$) but no difference was seen in the rate of SUI resolution ($P>.17$, percentages not reported). The investigators then examined the incremental effect of weight loss on SUI symptoms. Each kilogram of weight loss was associated with a 3% decrease in the odds of experiencing weekly SUI symptoms (odds ratio [OR] 0.97, 95% confidence interval [CI] 0.95–0.99, $P = .008$). Women who lost 5% to 10% of body weight were 33% less likely to report weekly SUI symptoms compared with women who maintained or gained (OR 0.67, 95% CI 0.47–0.95, $P = .03$). Those who lost 10% or more were 41% less likely to report symptoms (OR 0.59, 95% CI 0.40–0.87, $P = .008$).

Bladder Training

Bladder training is a noninvasive treatment that improves symptoms of urinary incontinence. Increased benefit is seen when training is supervised by a health care provider.

Bladder training consists of voiding at regularly scheduled intervals and using urge suppression techniques between voids, with a goal of decreasing total number of voids and incontinence episodes throughout the day. This common initial strategy for treatment of UUI was evaluated by Subak and colleagues[11] in an RCT of 123 women with urgency (38%), stress (24%), or mixed (37%) urinary incontinence. Women in the intervention group attended six 20-minute group instructional sessions on scheduled voiding and pelvic muscle exercises, and received individualized voiding schedules. The control group received no intervention. Women in the bladder training group reported a 50% decrease in leakage episodes on a 7-day voiding diary, compared with 15% in the controls ($P = .001$). Notably, results were not stratified by type of incontinence, limiting the ability to interpret the impact of bladder training on stress urinary leakage specifically.

Goode and colleagues[12] evaluated pelvic floor muscle training–based behavioral therapy in a multiarm RCT. Two-hundred women with SUI or MUI were randomly assigned to supervised behavioral training, supervised behavioral training combined with pelvic floor electrical stimulation (PFES), or to a control group of women who received a self-help booklet of behavioral training techniques. The behavioral training group had 4 biweekly visits with nurse practitioners, including biofeedback to teach correct performance of pelvic floor contractions and advance their exercise regimen. The PFES group was additionally provided a home PFES unit for use on alternating days. All patients, including the control group, were instructed to perform 3 sets of fifteen 2-second to 4-second pelvic floor muscle contractions daily, use preemptive contractions before leakage-promoting activities, and use urge suppression techniques (so-called freeze and squeeze). The primary outcome was reduction in incontinence episodes on bladder diary. Incontinence episodes were reduced by 69% with supervised behavioral training alone, 72% with the addition of PFES, and 53% for subjects who received a pelvic floor muscle exercise instruction booklet without supervision. Improvement in both the behavioral training and PFES groups were significantly higher compared with controls, but not different from each other ($P = .02$, $P = .002$, and $P = .60$).

Pelvic Floor Muscle Therapy Versus No Treatment

Physical therapy directed at improving pelvic muscle function is a long-standing primary treatment of SUI. In 1948, Kegel[13] reported improvement of incontinence symptoms in women using pelvic floor strengthening exercises. Over the subsequent half-century, instructions for pelvic muscle contractions have been supplemented with biofeedback devices, electrical stimulation, and weighted vaginal cones. PFMT as a treatment modality for SUI has been compared with both expectant and surgical management.

Supervised PFMT results in improvement in SUI symptoms with low risk of adverse events. However, absolute cure rates are low.

PFMT was compared with expectant management by Bø and colleagues[14] in 1999. In a multiarm design, 122 women with SUI were randomized to PFMT, daily use of vaginal electrical stimulation, daily use of weighted vaginal cones, or no treatment. Patients in the PFMT arm performed 3 daily sets of 8 to 12 high-intensity contractions lasting 6 to 8 seconds. Correct use of pelvic muscles was confirmed at enrollment by a physical therapist. The primary outcomes were change from baseline in pad weight on standardized stress test, and SUI symptoms on a 5-point scale from unproblematic to very problematic. At 6 months, pad weight decreased significantly more for women in the PFMT group compared with the other 3 groups (PFMT 30.2 g vs control 12.7 g, $P = .02$; electrical stimulation 7.4 g, $P = .02$; and vaginal cones 14.7 g, $P<.001$). Fifty-six percent of women reported that their incontinence was unproblematic after PFMT compared with 3% in controls, 12% following electrical stimulation, and 7% following vaginal cone use ($P<.001$). Pelvic floor muscle strength also improved significantly in the PFMT compared with the control group ($P<.01$).

The ability of PFMT to improve SUI symptoms was confirmed by a Cochrane systematic review and meta-analysis of trials comparing PFMT with no treatment, sham, or placebo.[15] Women who underwent PFMT for SUI were 8 times more likely to report cure (56.1% vs 6.0%; relative risk [RR] 8.38, 95% CI 3.68–19.07, based on 2 studies including 232 women) and 17 times more likely to report cure or improvement (55% vs 3.2%, RR 17.33, 95% CI 4.31–69.64 based on 4 studies of 260 women). PFMT was also associated with fewer leakage episodes per day and less urine loss on pad tests, and these patients were 5 times more likely to be satisfied with treatment (70.6% vs 12.9%, RR 5.32, 95% CI 2.63–10.74). Adverse events were rare and minor (pain, discomfort, or bother related to physical therapy).

Compared with PFMT, midurethral sling (MUS) surgery results in superior improvement in SUI but includes risks associated with surgery. Many women with moderate to severe SUI who initiate PFMT ultimately opt for surgical management and can expect comparable results.

Supervised PFMT was compared with MUS (**Fig. 1**) as primary treatment of moderate to severe SUI or stress-predominant MUI in a multicenter randomized controlled trial of 460 women.[16] PFMT entailed weekly or biweekly visits supervised by a certified pelvic floor physical therapist over 9 to 18 weeks, and included biofeedback or electrical stimulation at the discretion of the treating provider. The primary outcome was subjective improvement in symptoms (much or very much better) as measured by the Patient Global Impression of Improvement (PGI-I) scale. Subjective and objective cure were secondary outcomes, defined as an absence of SUI symptoms and negative cough stress test at 300 mL respectively. The study design allowed women to cross over from one treatment group to another if they were dissatisfied with the result

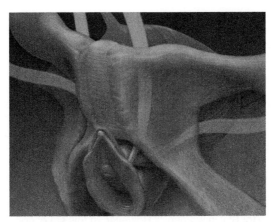

Fig. 1. Retropubic and transobturator MUS locations. (*Illustration copyright* Scott Bodell; with permission.)

of their treatment, and 49% of women initially randomized to PFMT opted for a MUS in the study, whereas 11.2% of women crossed over to PFMT after primary MUS. In the intention-to-treat analysis, subjective improvement in SUI symptoms at 12 months was 91% among women who were randomized to MUS, versus 65% following randomization to PFMT. Results were similar for women who underwent MUS as a primary treatment compared with those who crossed over after a trial of PFMT (91% vs 93%, $P = .68$). However, only 32% of women who received PFMT and did not cross over reported subjective improvement ($P<.001$). Subjective and objective cure rates were 85% and 77% for women who underwent initial surgery but only 16% and 44% for women who underwent PFMT ($P<.001$). Adverse events were exclusively reported in the surgery group and included bladder or vaginal trocar perforation, reoperation for urinary retention or mesh exposure, blood loss greater than 500 mL, hematoma, postoperative bleeding, and new urge urinary incontinence.

Pelvic Floor Muscle Therapy Versus Incontinence Pessary

Women seeking nonsurgical management for stress-predominant urinary incontinence can expect similar 1-year continence outcomes from an incontinence pessary or PFMT, provided a continence pessary can be satisfactorily fitted.

The most robust data on the effectiveness of and satisfaction with incontinence pessaries comes from the Ambulatory Treatments for Leakage Associated with Stress Incontinence (ATLAS) trial.[17] This multicenter trial randomized 446 women with SUI or stress-predominant MUI to an incontinence pessary, PFMT, or a combination of both. The 2 primary outcomes were subjective cure, defined as absence of retreatment and absence of bothersome SUI symptoms measured by Urogenital Distress Inventory, and subjective improvement in symptoms (much or very much better) as measured by the PGI-I scale.

The attrition rate of 26% in the pessary group was significantly higher than in the other 2 groups (15% and 12% for PFMT and combination group respectively; $P = .015$), primarily because of unsuccessful pessary fit (8%) and patient request for alternative treatment after randomization to pessary (7%). There were no differences in outcomes in the per protocol analysis of women successfully using each modality; subjective cure was 61%, 63%, and 41% for the pessary, PFMT, and combination arms respectively; and subjective improvement was 58%, 53%, and 44%

(P = nonsignificant [NS] for all). Patient satisfaction at 1 year ranged from 50% to 54% without differences between the groups when assessed based on initial group assignment. However, in the per protocol analysis, reported satisfaction rates were 91%, 87%, and 85% for pessary, PFMT, and combination group respectively (P = NS). Investigators concluded that success and satisfaction associated with the 2 nonsurgical management strategies for SUI were comparable contingent on a successful pessary fit. The investigators further concluded that combined therapy with pessary and PFMT did not offer any benefit compared with single therapy as first-line therapy, and that an incontinence pessary is an alternative to PFMT for patients who desire nonsurgical management and are unable to participate or access PFMT.

SURGICAL MANAGEMENT

The synthetic mesh MUS has been broadly adopted and is widely considered the gold standard procedure for SUI in women.[18] However, in this era of concern regarding the potential negative sequelae of mesh procedures, there has been a resurgence of interest in nonmesh SUI procedures among patients and providers. Evidence from comparative clinical trials investigating the MUS as well as nonmesh procedures is summarized later.

Retropubic Versus Transobturator Midurethral Sling

High-quality, long-term data with up to 5-year follow-up after retropubic and transobturator MUS show high and comparable satisfaction; subjective or objective continence outcomes are not significantly different, although adverse event profiles differ between approaches.

In a landmark study, the multicenter Trial of Midurethral Slings (TOMUS) randomized 597 women with stress-predominant urinary incontinence to retropubic MUS (RMUS) or transobturator MUS (TMUS) (see **Fig. 1**).[19] This was an equivalence trial, in which the two procedures would be considered equivalent if the postoperative success rates decreased to within a predetermined margin of ±12%. Objective success required a negative stress test, 24-hour pad test, and no SUI retreatment, whereas subjective success required absence of SUI symptoms, no leakage on a 3-day diary, and no retreatment. Both measures were primary outcomes and were reported at 12 and 24 months. Extended outcomes were reported at 5 years.

At 12 months, only objective success rate met the prespecified criteria for equivalence (RMUS vs. TMUS 80.8% vs. 77.7%, difference of 3.0% 95% CI −3.6% to 9.6%). At 24 months, neither objective nor subjective success rates met the equivalence criteria. Objective success rates at 24 months were 77.3% and 72.3% (difference 5.1%, 95% CI −2.0% to 12.1%) and subjective success rates were 55.7% and 48.3% (difference 7.4%, 95% CI −0.7% to 15.5%) for RMUS and TMUS respectively.[20] Because the CIs were outside the predetermined range of ±12% the two procedures could not be considered equivalent, but the CIs also include zero, indicating that the success rates are not significantly different from one another.

The definition of success was modified in the extended follow-up interval (up to 5 years after surgery) to be absence of retreatment and absence of SUI symptoms.[21] At that point, success rates for the two MUS routes did not meet equivalence criteria (RMUS vs TMUS 51.3% vs 43.4%, difference 7.9%, 95% CI −1.4% to 17.28%). Although the absolute success rates at each time point and by each definition were higher following RMUS, the differences were not statistically significant. The groups differed in their adverse event profile.[22]

Voiding dysfunction requiring surgical management and bladder perforations occurred exclusively in the RMUS group (3% and 5% vs 0.0%, $P<.001$ and $P = .002$), whereas neurologic symptoms (primarily pain) were twice as common following TMUS (5.4% vs 9.7%, $P = .04$). All bladder perforations were managed intraoperatively without clinically recognized sequelae through 12 months. Group rates of de novo and persistent urgency incontinence were comparable (RMUS vs TMUS, 0.0% vs 0.3%, $P>.99$, and 14.1% vs 12.8%, $P = .63$), mesh complications were similar and infrequent at 4.7% and 3% (RMUS and TMUS respectively). Importantly, patient satisfaction was high and similar for both MUS groups (RMUS vs TMUS, 86% vs 90%, $P = .52$) and adverse events had no effect on subjective or objective surgical success.[22,23]

Results from TOMUS and 20 additional RCTs comparing retropubic with transobturator MUS were summarized in the Society for Gynecologic Surgeons (SGS) systematic review and meta-analysis, incorporating data from more than 3000 women.[24] Meta-analysis favored RMUS for both objective and subjective cure rates; however, the findings were not statistically significant (OR 1.18, 95% CI 0.95–1.47; and OR 1.17, 95% CI 0.91–1.51). Overall satisfaction, reported in 4 studies, was comparable (OR 0.77, 95% CI 0.52–1.13). Overactive bladder (OAB) symptoms were more common following RMUS (OR 1.41, 95% CI 1.01–1.98, $P = .46$), whereas the reoperation rates did not differ for either retention or mesh erosion (RMUS vs TMUS, 1.2% vs 1.1% and 1.9% vs 2.7%; ORs not reported). Systematic review found groin pain to occur after 6.5% of TMUS versus 1.5% of RMUS, but meta-analysis was not performed for this outcome.

Fascial Pubovaginal Sling Versus Midurethral Slings

Retropubic MUS and fascial pubovaginal sling (PVS) result in similar rates of continence, reoperation for urinary retention, and de novo postoperative urgency symptoms. Retropubic MUS is a shorter procedure.

Outcomes after autologous fascial PVSs (**Fig. 2**) and retropubic MUSs were compared in five RCTs and a systematic review with metanalysis.[24,25] The studies are limited by small sample sizes and short follow-up. The largest trial randomized 100 women with urodynamic SUI and urethral hypermobility to RMUS or PVS.[25] Objective success measures were a negative full-bladder cough stress test and 1-hour pad test, and subjective success measures were International Incontinence Questionnaire (IIQ) score and patient satisfaction by visual analog scale (VAS). Short-term follow-up at 6 months found no differences in objective or subjective success (cough stress test 88% vs 83%, $P = .9$; pad test 75% vs 76%, $P = .83$; IIQ score 44.3 vs 48.5, $P = .05$; VAS ≥8 on a 10-point scale, 72% vs 55%, $P = .9$, RMUS vs PVS respectively). Rates of de novo urge incontinence and sling release were similar. The advantage of a MUS was shorter procedure time (45 vs 80 minutes, $P = .01$). Notably, 40% of the population had previously undergone incontinence surgery. In addition, these results have to be interpreted in the context of a moderate sample size, especially because this trial did not include a power calculation.

A systematic review and meta-analysis of studies comparing PVS and MUS were limited by small sample sizes and variable reporting of outcomes.[24] Meta-analysis favored MUS for subjective outcomes (OR 0.40, 95% CI 0.18–0.85) and found no group differences in adverse events overall, including postoperative overactive bladder symptoms (RMUS 6.9% vs PVS 8.6%), return to the operating room for urinary retention (1.2% vs 3%), or graft erosion (1.9% vs 1.6%).

Burch Colposuspension Versus Midurethral Sling

Open Burch colposuspension and MUS result in similar rates of continence, reoperation for urinary retention, and de novo postoperative urgency symptoms. MUS is a

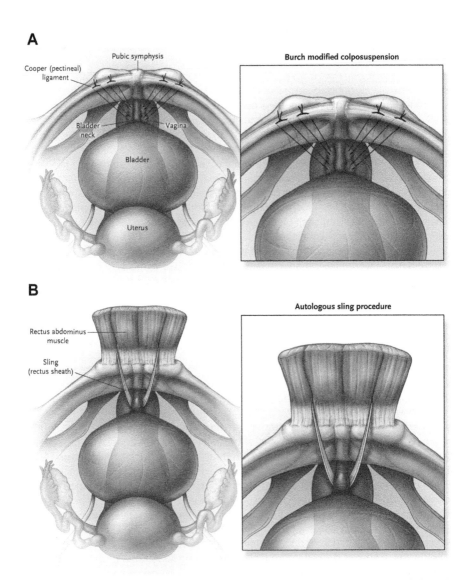

Fig. 2. Burch modified colposuspension (*A*) and autologous fascial pubovaginal sling (*B*) procedures. (*From* Albo ME, Richter HE, Brubaker L, et al. Burch colposuspension versus fascial sling to reduce urinary stress incontinence. N Engl J Med 2007;356:2143–55; and *Courtesy of* Massachusetts Medical Society, Waltham (MA); with permission.)

shorter procedure. Laparoscopic Burch results in lower objective cure rates compared with MUS, but subjective results are similar.

There are 7 RCTs and 2 systematic reviews comparing open Burch colposuspension (see **Fig. 2**) and synthetic MUS.[24,26,27] The largest multicenter RCT, by Ward and colleagues,[27] randomized 315 women with urodynamic SUI and no detrusor overactivity to either retropubic MUS or to open Burch colposuspension. Their primary outcome was a composite objective measure of negative urodynamic stress test and 1-hour pad test. Subjective cure, ascertained by the Bristol Female Lower Urinary

Tract Symptoms questionnaire was a secondary outcome. The investigators found no significant difference in objective or subjective cure rates between synthetic mesh midurethral slings and Burch colposuspension at their primary end point of 6 months (66% vs 57%, P = .099; and 59% vs 53%, P = NS). Cure rates remained similar between groups at 2-year and 5-year follow-up, with negative 1-hour pad tests in 81% and 80% at 2 years, although study attrition exceeded 50% by 5 years.[28,29] Surgical retreatment of persistent SUI was low and not different between groups (3.4% vs 1.8% for the Burch and RMUS groups respectively). Notably, the study was limited by early recruitment termination, resulting in insufficient power to detect potential differences, and a disproportionate attrition before assigned surgery in the Burch group, which compromised the baseline equivalence of the two groups.

A Cochrane Review of 6 trials has similarly reported equivalent success rates between open Burch and synthetic MUS (82% and 79% respectively).[26] Rates of de novo urgency or urgency incontinence, and surgical retreatment of persistent incontinence, were also similar after Burch and MUS (13% vs 9%, RR 0.69, 95% CI 0.38–1.24; and RR 0.52, 95% CI 0.13–2.12, respectively). MUSs were on average 15.5 minutes shorter but were associated with more bladder perforations (6% vs 1%, RR 4.24, 95% CI 1.71–10.52).

Clinical outcomes after minimally invasive laparoscopic Burch and synthetic mesh MUS have been reported in 8 studies. The Cochrane group found that objective outcomes favored MUS when compared with laparoscopic Burch by a small margin (RR 0.88, 95% CI 0.81–0.95), whereas subjective cure rates appeared equivalent (RR 0.91, 95% CI 0.80–1.02), as did the rates of perioperative complications and de novo detrusor overactivity. Procedure time was on average 20 minutes longer in the laparoscopic Burch group.

The comparable continence outcomes after open Burch and MUS procedures were reiterated in the systematic review and meta-analysis conducted by the Society for Gynecologic Surgeons.[24] The comparison of MUS with Burch included 10 studies, incorporating RMUS (8 studies) TMUS (2 studies), open Burch (7 studies), and laparoscopic Burch (3 studies). The meta-analysis found no significant difference in objective or subjective cure rates, occurrence of postoperative OAB symptoms, or return to the operating room for either erosion or retention. On systematic review, absolute rates of wound infection were higher following Burch procedures (Burch 7%, RMUS 0.74%, TMUS 0.75%). Rate of retreatment of persistent incontinence was not summarized.

Fascial Pubovaginal Slings Versus Burch Colposuspension

Fascial PVSs result in higher continence rates, improved patient satisfaction, and lower rates of repeat incontinence surgery compared with Burch colposuspension, but are associated with more postoperative voiding dysfunction and urinary retention.

The autologous fascial PVS was compared with open Burch colposuspension in the Stress Incontinence Surgical Treatment Efficacy Trial (SISTEr), a multicenter randomized trial of 655 women with demonstrable SUI or stress-predominant MUI and urethral hypermobility.[30] Concomitant prolapse surgeries were permitted. There were 2 primary outcomes: a composite measure of stress incontinence cure, and a composite measure of overall cure. Cure of SUI was defined as absence of SUI symptoms, no retreatment of SUI, and a negative stress test. Overall cure criteria additionally included no leakage on a 3-day diary, pad weight increase of less than 15 g on a 24-hour test, and absence of symptoms or retreatment of any type of incontinence. At 2 years, women who underwent sling surgery had higher stress-specific and overall cure rates (66% vs 49%, $P<.001$; and 47% vs 38%, P = .01 for autologous sling and Burch colposuspension respectively). This superiority among sling recipients persisted throughout 5 years of follow-up, although success rates diminished to 31% and 24% by the study's stringent criteria.[31] Notably, the investigators postulated that these 5-year success rates reflect bias toward failure, because 85% of women reporting failure at the 2-year end point agreed to extended follow-up, compared with only 52% of women reporting treatment success. Patient satisfaction correlated with continence status and was highest among the sling group at both 2-year and 5-year follow-up (86% vs 78%, $P = .02$; and 83% vs 73%, $P = .04$). The SISTEr surgical groups had significantly different adverse event profiles.[32] Sling surgery was associated with more urinary retention leading to a 6% reoperation rate for retention or voiding symptoms (vs 0% following Burch), whereas 11% of women in the Burch group pursued surgical retreatment of persistent incontinence (vs 2% following sling; $P<.001$).

Full-length Midurethral Slings Versus Single-incision Minislings

At present, available minislings and full-length transobturator MUSs result in similar short-term continence rates, but long-term data are lacking. It is yet to be determined whether minislings offer a clinically meaningful advantage.

The newest modification to MUS is the minisling or single-incision sling, which requires only a vaginal incision and does not pass through the retropubic space or the obturator foramen. Purported advantages of these products include less pain and reduced visceral injuries or other perioperative complications compared with full-length MUS. The SGS systematic review and meta-analysis identified 15 trials comparing full-length MUS with minislings, 13 of which evaluated the TVT-Secure, which has subsequently been withdrawn from the market.[24] However, TVT-Secure data were included because there were otherwise insufficient data for analysis. Meta-analysis showed superior subjective and objective success rates with full-length MUS slings compared with minislings (OR 2.65, 95% CI 1.36–5.17; and OR 4.16, 95% CI 2.05–6.08). The investigators did not identify a clear advantage in terms of overall adverse events.

Since that publication, other studies comparing minisling products with full-length transobturator MUSs have reported comparable short-term outcomes. An industry-sponsored, multicenter, randomized, noninferiority trial of 193 women with SUI to MiniArc or Monarc MUS (American Medical Systems, Minneapolis, MN) with a primary outcome of subjective success defined by much or very much improved on PGI-I found no group differences at 12 months (83% and 86%, Monarc MUS and MiniArc respectively, $P = .46$).[33] Patients who underwent MiniArc reported less pain in the first 3 days postoperatively as measured by VAS from 0 to 100 (mean VAS score 9 vs 22, $P<.01$), experienced less blood loss (20 vs 50 mL, $P<.01$) and shorter operative time (10 vs 15 minutes, $P<.01$). The clinical impact of these differences was not established.

Similarly, Lee and colleagues[34] reported comparable 12-month objective success rates, defined as negative cough stress test in an RCT comparing MiniArc and Monarc among 215 women with SUI (92.2% vs 94.2%, $P = .78$, difference 2.0%, 95% CI −2.7% to 6.7%). Subjective success was also similar (94.4% vs 96.7%, $P = .50$, difference 2.3%, 95% CI −1.5% to +6.1%).

Periurethral Bulking Injections

Small, randomized studies suggest superior improvement in SUI symptoms following bulking compared with unsupervised pelvic floor muscle strengthening, but an inferior outcome compared with PVS.

Bulking agents can be injected adjacent to the urethra via a transurethral or periurethral approach in an ambulatory setting with minimal anesthesia, and offer an alternative low-risk, nonmesh strategy for women with SUI. Counseling regarding expected outcomes from bulking agent injection is hampered by minimal data to guide selection of appropriate patients, injectable agent, or route of injection. At present, available agents in the United States are Macroplastique (Cogentix, Minnetonka, MN), a silicone polymer in a carrier gel, and Coaptite (BioForm Medical Inc, Franksville, WI), which contains calcium hydroxylapatite particles in an aqueous gel. Contigen (Bard, Murray Hill, NJ), glutaraldehyde cross-linked bovine collagen, was US Food and Drug Administration approved in 1993. It was a widely used agent until the manufacturer ceased production in 2011.

There are no published studies that have compared the available bulking agents with a control. Therefore, no conclusions can be made regarding the efficacy of contemporary bulking therapy compared with expectant management of SUI symptoms. There are no published trials comparing available bulking agents, or routes of injection.

Transurethral Macroplastique injection was compared with a control treatment of written instructions for home-based pelvic floor strengthening in a small RCT of 45 women with urodynamic SUI and urethral hypermobility.[35] Sixty-three percent of Macroplastique recipients reported that their symptoms were cured or markedly improved at 3 months, whereas 21% underwent a repeat bulking injection at 3 months because of treatment failure. Among controls, only 9% reported cure or marked improvement (*P* value not reported). Adverse events were only reported in the Macroplastique group, and included a 74% rate of urinary retention and 47% rate of postoperative dysuria.

Another small trial randomized 45 women with SUI and intrinsic sphincter deficiency to PVS or Macroplastique.[36] Urodynamic cure at 6 months was 81% following PVS, compared with 9% following Macroplastique (*P*<.001), and 31% of bulking patients pursued further surgery versus 5% following PVS (*P* value not reported).

SUMMARY

Women seeking relief from symptoms of SUI have a broad array of treatment options ranging from lifestyle modification to surgical interventions, with differing effectiveness and associated risk. Providers and patient can use information from clinical trials to develop individualized treatment plans oriented to a woman's lifestyle, expectations and goals for treatment, as well as her tolerance for potential adverse events.

REFERENCES

1. Nygaard I, Barber MD, Burgio KL, et al. Prevalence of symptomatic pelvic floor disorders in US women. JAMA 2008;300(11):1311–6.
2. Fultz NH, Burgio K, Diokno AC, et al. Burden of stress urinary incontinence for community-dwelling women. Am J Obstet Gynecol 2003;189(5):1275–82.
3. Hampel C, Wienhold D, Benken N, et al. Definition of overactive bladder and epidemiology of urinary incontinence. Urology 1997;50(6A Suppl):4–14 [discussion: 15–7].
4. Abrams P, Cardozo L, Fall M, et al. The standardisation of terminology of lower urinary tract function: report from the Standardisation Sub-committee of the International Continence Society. Am J Obstet Gynecol 2002;187(1):116–26.
5. Wu JM, Matthews CA, Conover MM, et al. Lifetime risk of stress urinary incontinence or pelvic organ prolapse surgery. Obstet Gynecol 2014;123(6):1201–6.
6. Alling Moller L, Lose G, Jorgensen T. Risk factors for lower urinary tract symptoms in women 40 to 60 years of age. Obstet Gynecol 2000;96(3):446–51.

7. Danforth KN, Townsend MK, Lifford K, et al. Risk factors for urinary incontinence among middle-aged women. Am J Obstet Gynecol 2006;194(2):339–45.
8. Subak LL, Wing R, West DS, et al. Weight loss to treat urinary incontinence in overweight and obese women. N Engl J Med 2009;360(5):481–90.
9. Wing RR, Creasman JM, West DS, et al. Improving urinary incontinence in overweight and obese women through modest weight loss. Obstet Gynecol 2010; 116(2 Pt 1):284–92.
10. Phelan S, Kanaya AM, Subak LL, et al. Weight loss prevents urinary incontinence in women with type 2 diabetes: results from the Look AHEAD trial. J Urol 2012; 187(3):939–44.
11. Subak LL, Quesenberry CP, Posner SF, et al. The effect of behavioral therapy on urinary incontinence: a randomized controlled trial. Obstet Gynecol 2002;100(1): 72–8.
12. Goode PS, Burgio KL, Locher JL, et al. Effect of behavioral training with or without pelvic floor electrical stimulation on stress incontinence in women: a randomized controlled trial. JAMA 2003;290(3):345–52.
13. Kegel AH. Progressive resistance exercise in the functional restoration of the perineal muscles. Am J Obstet Gynecol 1948;56(2):238–48.
14. Bø K, Talseth T, Holme I. Single blind, randomised controlled trial of pelvic floor exercises, electrical stimulation, vaginal cones, and no treatment in management of genuine stress incontinence in women. BMJ 1999;318:487–93.
15. Dumoulin C, Hay-Smith EJ, Mac Habee-Seguin G. Pelvic floor muscle training versus no treatment, or inactive control treatments, for urinary incontinence in women. Cochrane Database Syst Rev 2014;(5):CD005654.
16. Labrie J, Berghmans BL, Fischer K, et al. Surgery versus physiotherapy for stress urinary incontinence. N Engl J Med 2013;369(12):1124–33.
17. Richter HE, Burgio KL, Brubaker L, et al. Continence pessary compared with behavioral therapy or combined therapy for stress incontinence: a randomized controlled trial. Obstet Gynecol 2010;115(3):609–17.
18. Cox A, Herschorn S, Lee L. Surgical management of female SUI: is there a gold standard? Nat Rev Urol 2013;10(2):78–89.
19. Richter HE, Albo ME, Zyczynski HM, et al. Retropubic versus transobturator midurethral slings for stress incontinence. N Engl J Med 2010;362(22):2066–76.
20. Albo ME, Litman HJ, Richter HE, et al. Treatment success of retropubic and transobturator mid urethral slings at 24 months. J Urol 2012;188(6):2281–7.
21. Kenton K, Stoddard AM, Zyczynski H, et al. 5-year longitudinal followup after retropubic and transobturator mid urethral slings. J Urol 2015;193(1):203–10.
22. Brubaker L, Norton PA, Albo ME, et al. Adverse events over two years after retropubic or transobturator midurethral sling surgery: findings from the Trial of Midurethral Slings (TOMUS) study. Am J Obstet Gynecol 2011;205(5):498.e1–6.
23. Wai CY, Curto TM, Zyczynski HM, et al. Patient satisfaction after midurethral sling surgery for stress urinary incontinence. Obstet Gynecol 2013;121(5):1009–16.
24. Schimpf MO, Rahn DD, Wheeler TL, et al. Sling surgery for stress urinary incontinence in women: a systematic review and metaanalysis. Am J Obstet Gynecol 2014;211(1):71.e1–27.
25. Sharifiaghdas F, Mortazavi N. Tension-free vaginal tape and autologous rectus fascia pubovaginal sling for the treatment of urinary stress incontinence: a medium-term follow-up. Med Princ Pract 2008;17(3):209–14.
26. Ogah J, Cody JD, Rogerson L. Minimally invasive synthetic suburethral sling operations for stress urinary incontinence in women. Cochrane Database Syst Rev 2009;(4):CD006375.

27. Ward K, Hilton P, United Kingdom and Ireland Tension-free Vaginal Tape Trial Group. Prospective multicentre randomised trial of tension-free vaginal tape and colposuspension as primary treatment for stress incontinence. BMJ 2002; 325(7355):67.
28. Ward KL, Hilton P, UK and Ireland TVT Trial Group. A prospective multicenter randomized trial of tension-free vaginal tape and colposuspension for primary urodynamic stress incontinence: two-year follow-up. Am J Obstet Gynecol 2004; 190(2):324–31.
29. Ward KL, Hilton P, UK and Ireland TVT Trial Group. Tension-free vaginal tape versus colposuspension for primary urodynamic stress incontinence: 5-year follow up. BJOG 2008;115(2):226–33.
30. Albo ME, Richter HE, Brubaker L, et al. Burch colposuspension versus fascial sling to reduce urinary stress incontinence. N Engl J Med 2007;356(21):2143–55.
31. Brubaker L, Richter HE, Norton PA, et al. 5-year continence rates, satisfaction and adverse events of Burch urethropexy and fascial sling surgery for urinary incontinence. J Urol 2012;187(4):1324–30.
32. Chai TC, Albo ME, Richter HE, et al. Complications in women undergoing Burch colposuspension versus autologous rectus fascial sling for stress urinary incontinence. J Urol 2009;181(5):2192–7.
33. Schellart RP, Oude Rengerink K, Van der Aa F, et al. A randomized comparison of a single-incision midurethral sling and a transobturator midurethral sling in women with stress urinary incontinence: results of 12-mo follow-up. Eur Urol 2014;66(6):1179–85.
34. Lee JK, Rosamilia A, Dwyer PL, et al. Randomized trial of a single incision versus an outside-in transobturator midurethral sling in women with stress urinary incontinence: 12 month results. Am J Obstet Gynecol 2015;213(1):35.e1–9.
35. ter Meulen PH, Berghmans LC, Nieman FH, et al. Effects of Macroplastique Implantation System for stress urinary incontinence and urethral hypermobility in women. Int Urogynecol J Pelvic Floor Dysfunct 2009;20(2):177–83.
36. Maher CF, O'Reilly BA, Dwyer PL, et al. Pubovaginal sling versus transurethral Macroplastique for stress urinary incontinence and intrinsic sphincter deficiency: a prospective randomised controlled trial. BJOG 2005;112(6):797–801.

Overactive Bladder

Nicola White, MD[a], Cheryl B. Iglesia, MD[b,c],*

KEYWORDS

- Overactive bladder • Urinary incontinence
- Bladder botulinum toxin (Botox) injection • Anticholinergics
- Sacral neuromodulation

KEY POINTS

- Overactive bladder is a syndrome affecting millions of women worldwide and prevalence will increase as the population ages.
- Pelvic floor physical therapy or muscle retraining is considered first-line treatment and has demonstrated improvement in OAB symptoms when compared with no intervention with no adverse outcomes; however, more data are needed on long-term effectiveness.
- Anticholinergic therapy is currently a mainstay of therapy but is often discontinued due to side effects and inefficacy.
- Newer therapies such as intradetrusor injection of onabotulinum toxin and neuromodulation (via percutaneous tibial nerve and implanted direct sacral nerve stimulation) have shown promising results as viable treatment alternatives to anticholinergic therapy treatment for overactive bladder.
- Further research is needed to compare long-term efficacy, side effects/adverse events and cost-effectiveness of the multiple available treatment options for overactive bladder.

INTRODUCTION

Overactive bladder (OAB) is a syndrome defined by the International Continence Society as "urinary urgency, usually accompanied by frequency and nocturia, with or without urgency urinary incontinence (UI), in the absence of urinary tract infection (UTI) or other obvious pathology." OAB occurs with or without incontinence, referred

[a] Female Pelvic Medicine and Reconstructive Surgery, National Center for Advanced Pelvic Surgery, MedStar Washington Hospital Center, Georgetown University, 106 Irving Street, Northwest, Suite 405 South, Washington, DC 20010, USA; [b] Section of Female Pelvic Medicine and Reconstructive Surgery, Department of Obstetrics and Gynecology, MedStar Washington Hospital Center, Georgetown University School of Medicine, 106 Irving Street, Northwest, Suite 405 South, Washington, DC 20010, USA; [c] Section of Female Pelvic Medicine and Reconstructive Surgery, Department of Urology, MedStar Washington Hospital Center, Georgetown University School of Medicine, 106 Irving Street, Northwest, Suite 405 South, Washington, DC 20010, USA
* Corresponding author. Section of Female Pelvic Medicine and Reconstructive Surgery, Department of Obstetrics and Gynecology, MedStar Washington Hospital Center, Georgetown University School of Medicine, 106 Irving Street, Northwest, Suite 405 South, Washington, DC 20010.
E-mail address: Cheryl.iglesia@medstar.net

Obstet Gynecol Clin N Am 43 (2016) 59–68
http://dx.doi.org/10.1016/j.ogc.2015.10.002
0889-8545/16/$ – see front matter © 2016 Elsevier Inc. All rights reserved.

obgyn.theclinics.com

to as OAB (wet) and OAB (dry), respectively. Approximately two-thirds of patients reporting symptoms of urgency and frequency do not have concurrent incontinence (*OAB* dry), whereas one-third do experience incontinence with their symptoms (*OAB* wet).

Heterogeneity in symptoms and underreporting of symptoms by patients make the prevalence and incidence of overactive bladder difficult to establish. The NOBLE Program in 2001 used telephone surveys to ascertain the prevalence of OAB and found prevalence in the United States to be 16.9% in women, with slightly more than one-third of these women having incontinence associated with their OAB.[1] Prevalence of symptoms also increased with age. Another review showed a slighter higher rate of 18.6% for patients reporting these symptoms "often," with 28.7% of the adult US population reporting occasional ("sometimes") OAB symptoms.[2,3]

With the increasing age of the population in the United States and the high prevalence of this condition, overactive bladder represents a condition with a large economic impact. Estimates indicate that the adult US population spent an additional $24.9 billion per year to manage their urinary symptoms with much of this expenditure, in particular among institutionalized adults, related to incontinence products (eg, pads).[2] Estimates from more than 10 years ago indicate that women aged 60 to 80 are the largest growing segment of the population in the United States, so these estimates of costs are likely to increase significantly.

ETIOLOGY OF OVERACTIVE BLADDER

The cause of overactive bladder is not well understood but is thought to be multifactorial in nature. The lower urinary tract has 2 main functions: storage and elimination. A system of neurotransmitters through both autonomic and somatic pathways controls the balance between these 2 functions. Detrusor overactivity, defined by the International Continence Society as "involuntary detrusor contractions that may be spontaneous or provoked," as observed on urodynamics,[4] leads to overactive bladder, with or without incontinence. Approximately 90% of detrusor overactivity leading to symptoms of urgency and frequency with or without incontinence is idiopathic, without a recognizable etiology. However, a variety of neurologic, lower urinary tract anatomic abnormalities and other disorders can cause and/or exacerbate detrusor overactivity.

DIAGNOSIS OF OVERACTIVE BLADDER

Overactive bladder is a common condition that greatly impacts quality of life, and evaluation of the patient should start with an assessment of the degree to which the condition impacts the patient's daily life. Standardized quality-of-life questionnaires are available for use in evaluation. Additionally, taking a thorough medical and surgical history and a complete review of medications is vital to understanding an individual patient's experience with OAB.

Physical examination can elucidate underlying medical conditions contributing to symptoms. The examination should include a general physical examination, with special attention to the neurologic and pelvic examinations. Spinal cord segments S2 to S4 are involved in micturition and should be evaluated accordingly. Pelvic examination should assess for signs of atrophy, pelvic organ prolapse, pelvic floor muscle strength assessment, and any anatomic abnormalities, including urethral diverticulum.

Relevant laboratory testing includes urinalysis and possibly urine cytology if irritative bladder symptoms and significant microhematuria are present on urinalysis. UTI and chronic irritative bladder conditions can present like OAB. Measurement of postvoid residual volume (typically <150 mL) can help rule out overflow incontinence.

Urodynamic testing may be indicated to further investigate overactive bladder symptoms in patients with refractory symptoms, previous pelvic reconstructive surgery including anti-incontinence operations, neurologic diseases, or voiding dysfunction. Urodynamic testing starts with uninstrumented uroflowmetry (measuring flow rate and voiding time) followed by cystometry to assess bladder storage function during filling through a catheter to objectively diagnose detrusor overactivity as evidenced by uninhibited bladder contractions associated with urgency. In women with any concern for an underlying neurologic cause for OAB, electromyography (EMG) can be useful to evaluate activity of the external striated urethral sphincter muscles. EMG can evaluate whether a patient demonstrates coordination between the external sphincter which should relax when the detrusor muscle contracts and failure to do so may represent dyssynergic activity, indicating a possible upper motor neuron process.

MANAGEMENT OF OVERACTIVE BLADDER

The management of overactive bladder includes treating any underlying reversible medical conditions contributing to the syndrome, such as use of antibiotics for bladder infections, intervening for stress UI via surgery, weight loss or medical management, and optimizing glucose control in diabetes, with the goal of moving toward treatments targeted at specific bladder symptoms. A wide variety of behavioral interventions, pharmacologic agents, and more invasive options exists for treatment of OAB.

Behavioral Modifications and Pelvic Floor Muscle Retraining/Physical Therapy

One of the first behavioral interventions typically used in improving symptoms of OAB is bladder retraining. The American Urological Association (AUA)/Society for Urodynamics, Female Pelvic Medicine and Urogenital Reconstruction (SUFU) guidelines for non-neurogenic OAB in adults published in 2014 supports behavioral modifications as the recommended first-line treatment, based on current available evidence.[5] This process involves patient education on effects of caffeine and fluid intake and bowel function on symptoms and then works on scheduled voiding. A program is developed to increase intervals between voids to attempt to suppress urgency and decrease incontinence episodes. The theory behind pelvic floor muscle retraining for urge UI is based on the observation that a detrusor contraction can be inhibited by pelvic floor muscle contraction. Increasing the strength of the pelvic floor and ability of an individual to hold a contraction can result in extra time (perhaps just a few more seconds) to reach the toilet and avoid leakage.

A recent Cochrane review published in 2014 evaluated the effects of pelvic floor muscle retraining (PFMT) in UI, both stress and urge incontinence. No randomized controlled studies looked at urge incontinence only and the effects of PFMT. In the 3 trials including women with all types of UI, all reported that PFMT was better than the control group for complete resolution of symptoms.[6] However, in the study with a larger proportion of women specifically with urge incontinence, the rates of cure were reported as lower. All 3 of the studies reviewed showed a trend toward improved quality of life compared with no treatment. Further research into long-term effectiveness and cost-effectiveness for PFMT is warranted. Existing evidence is insufficient to make any strong recommendations about the best approach to PFMT. The therapy is not standardized nor monitored. Additionally, benefits to using pelvic floor physical therapy in combination with biofeedback has been shown to decrease symptoms of OAB, but these interventions do not maintain their effects at 15 years and can be difficult routines for patients to maintain over the long term.[7] Although specific trials for urge incontinence/overactive bladder symptoms and PFMT are needed, the evidence overall supports the use of pelvic floor muscle therapy as a first-line treatment for symptoms.

Medications

For many years, antimuscarinic medications have been used for treatment of OAB symptoms and are currently recommended by the AUA as the second-line treatment. Although there are 5 subtypes, the muscarinic receptors within the bladder are primarily of the M2 and M3 subtypes. When stimulated, the M2 receptor acts to inhibit the sympathetic pathways to the bladder, thereby inhibiting relaxation of the detrusor muscle. Once activated, the M3 receptors promote detrusor contractions. Antimuscarinic agents (also called anticholinergics) have been developed to act on these 2 receptors specifically.

A systematic review of the literature completed in 2012 for the Agency for Healthcare Research and Quality examined all the diagnostic studies and therapeutic randomized and nonrandomized studies published in English up to that time so as to determine efficacy and comparative effectiveness among pharmacologic treatments for UI. This study reported that benefits (defined as less perceived urgency and continence) were achieved with antimuscarinic drugs, including trospium, solifenacin, fesoterodine, tolterodine, and oxybutynin. Drugs for urgency UI demonstrated similar effectiveness. Treatment discontinuation due to adverse effects was most common with oxybutynin and least common with solifenacin. Common side effects include dry mouth, constipation, and blurred vision. Anticholinergics are contraindicated in patients with narrow-angle glaucoma and also carry the risk of urinary retention and should be used with caution in individuals with a degree of bladder outlet obstruction. All anticholinergic medications were more effective than placebo in achieving continence and improving UI, but the degree of benefit was low for all drugs.[8]

Similarly, Madhuvrata and colleagues[9] in a Cochrane review in 2012 reviewed the literature to compare specific formulations of anticholinergics. Oxybutynin and tolterodine are the 2 oldest drugs and, therefore, the most studied. Efficacy is similar but oxybutynin is discontinued more frequently secondary to side effects. Extended release formulations for both drugs carry fewer side effects. Solifenacin and fesoterodine were shown to be more effective than tolterodine.

The bladder contains both alpha-adrenergic and beta-adrenergic receptors and stimulation of these receptors can exert some influence on the bladder and urethra. Alpha-adrenergic agonists (ephedrine, phenylpropanolamine, pseudoephedrine) increase urethral pressure to decrease incontinence. Beta-adrenergic agonists (isoproterenol and terbutaline) result in bladder relaxation and decrease intravesical pressure. However, neither of these alpha-adrenergic or beta-adrenergic agonists has proven to be more effective than placebo.[10]

More recently, the Food and Drug Administration (FDA) approved the use of mirabegron for the treatment of OAB. Mirabegron is a β3-adrenergic agonist that acts specifically on the β3-adrenoreceptors in the wall of the bladder, causing wall relaxation during the filling and storage phase of micturition. Mirabegron was found in 3 separate randomized controlled clinical trials to significantly decrease urinary frequency and incontinence episodes, while significantly increasing bladder capacity.[11–13] Mirabegron has fewer reported side effects than anticholinergics but adverse effects include hypertension, nasopharyngitis, UTI, and headache. Patients on mirabegron should have their blood pressure monitored and it is contraindicated in patients with uncontrolled hypertension. Similar to anticholinergics, β3-adrenergic agonists can increase the risk for urinary retention so should be used with caution in patients with clinically significant bladder outlet obstruction.

Anticholinergics have a high rate of discontinuation due to side effects. There is a high discontinuation rate with only 18% of patients continuing with antimuscarinic medication after 6 months.[14] The extended release formulations and newer medications like the β3-adrenergic agonist mirabegron are better tolerated, but long-term use continues to be problematic.

Botulinum Toxin

In 2011, the FDA approved the use of bladder onabotulinumtoxinA (Botox A) injections into the bladder mucosa for treatment of neurogenic bladder and in 2013, it was approved for treatment of overactive bladder. Botulinum toxin has been FDA approved for other conditions, such as blepharospasm, and works on the bladder in a similar mechanism. The toxin acts a muscle paralytic by inhibiting the presynaptic release of acetylcholine from the motor neurons, thereby inhibiting muscle contraction. Botox A is injected in small aliquots directly into the bladder wall muscle (total 200 units injected at 30 sites for neurogenic bladder and total 100 units injected at 20 sites for OAB).

A Cochrane review published in 2011 looked at the results of Botox A use in 19 different studies, mostly treating neurogenic OAB, but several for treatment of idiopathic OAB. All 19 studies demonstrated improvement in symptoms using Botox injections compared with placebo. The EMBARK trial (randomized controlled trial [RCT] comparing Botox with placebo) showed a decrease in the daily frequency of UI episodes versus placebo (-2.65 vs -0.87, $P<0.001$) and 22.9% versus 6.5% of patients became completely continent. OnabotulinumtoxinA improved patient health-related quality of life across multiple measures ($P<0.001$).[15] The Cochrane review also found that higher doses (300 units) were found to be more effective but had more associated side effects, specifically urinary retention. The review also evaluated method of injection and determined that suburothelial injection had similar efficacy to intradetrusor injections. In terms of dosage, the data revealed that the length of effect of the toxin varies among patients and is dose-dependent. Patients receiving multiple doses did not appear to become refractory.[16]

The ABC trial by Visco and colleagues[17] for the Pelvic Floor Disorders Network was a double-blinded RCT comparing anticholinergic therapy to bladder botulinum toxin injections. Women assigned to the anticholinergic arm were allowed to increase dose of medication and change to a different anticholinergic depending on their symptom control, which mimics common practice. Anticholinergics and Botox injections were shown to have similar reductions in number of urge incontinence episodes daily; anticholinergics decreased 5.0 to 3.4 and Botox decreased 5.0 to 3.3. Complete resolution of symptoms occurred in 13% of patients in the anticholinergic arm and 27% of the patients who received Botox. Both therapies had similar levels of improvement on quality of life measurements. Anticholinergics were associated with greater rates of dry mouth and Botox had higher rates of voiding difficulty requiring intermittent self-catheterization and UTIs.

OnabotulinumtoxinA has an acceptable safety profile. Most common adverse effects include UTIs and urinary retention requiring self-catheterization (typically short term). The rate of UTI ranges from 2% to 32%.[18] UTIs are often associated with higher residual volumes. Several studies have shown increased risk of de novo need for self-catheterization (ISC) with higher doses of toxin injected. Popat and colleagues[19] reported a de novo risk of ISC of 69% with injection of 300 units and 19% with injection of 200 units. The ABC trial reported a rate of 5% for ISC with use of 100 units injected into the bladder detrusor muscle.[17] Systemic reactions including spasticity or chronic pain are extremely rare events with bladder injection of Botox.

Per the AUA/SUFU guidelines from 2014, Botox injections for OAB are considered third-line treatment for patients who have failed first-line (behavioral modifications) and second-line treatment (antimuscarinic medications) or are not candidates for anticholinergic medications.[5] Patients have to be willing to undergo the procedure and accept the risk of possible need for intermittent self-catheterization. Overall, review of the literature available for use of Botox for overactive bladder shows that Botox has an average duration of effect of 6 to 9 months. The duration of effect is both patient-dependent and dose-dependent. Higher doses (200–300 un) come with higher rates of retention. A meta-analysis of studies that followed patients using Botox long-term showed no loss of efficacy for up to 10 years of treatment and no decrease in effect of or development of intolerance.[18] Schmid and colleagues[20] showed that among patients with idiopathic detrusor overactivity, poor responders to Botox were more likely to have low pretreatment detrusor compliance (<10 mL/cm H2O) and a maximum bladder capacity of less than 100 mL. These results were similar to findings reported by Compérat and colleagues[21] for neurogenic detrusor activity.

The available research on Botox intradetrusor injections overall supports its use for overactive bladder symptoms. The data show a decrease in the bothersome symptoms of incontinence and urinary frequency. Although the risk of urinary retention causing UTI or need for self-catheterization is low, it remains an important risk factor to discuss with patients. Long-term data support its continued use, but patients also must be aware that repeat injections are to be expected.

Percutaneous Tibial Nerve Stimulation

Percutaneous tibial nerve stimulation (PTNS) is a minimally invasive, outpatient treatment that has been shown to decrease symptoms related to OAB. The procedure involves placing a small needle electrode into the lower inner aspect of either leg near the medial malleolus. The electrode is connected to a stimulator that generates an electrical pulse, which then travels to the sacral nerve plexus via the tibial nerve. The treatment course involves 12 weekly 30-minute sessions, sometimes requiring monthly maintenance session. The procedure is not painful and no side effects have been shown. Similar to sacral neuromodulation, accessing the posterior tibial nerve stimulates sensory afferent nerves, but PTNS does so in a less-invasive manner compared with direct sacral neuromodulation.

Three RCTs have been published for the treatment of overactive bladder with percutaneous nerve stimulation. The reported rates of success for PTNS were variable (54.5%–79.5%) for treating OAB symptoms among these trials.[22] Another meta-analysis by Burton and colleagues[23] found that patients who received PTNS were 7 times more likely to have successful treatment compared with placebo. Peters and colleagues[24] developed a sham procedure and performed an RCT comparing PTNS to the sham procedure. They reported a statistically significant improvement in bladder symptoms with 54.5% of patients receiving PTNS reporting moderately or markedly improved responses compared with 20.9% of sham subjects from baseline (P<.001). Peters and colleagues[25] also performed an RCT comparing PTNS to tolterodine 4 mg extended release and showed a statistically significant improvement in OAB symptoms in the PTNS group compared with the sham procedure group

(79.5% reporting cure or improvement vs 54.8%, $P = .01$). Additionally, Finazzi-Agrò and colleagues[26] undertook a prospective, double-blinded RCT comparing PTNS with placebo and found that 71% of those in the PTNS group were considered "responders" to treatment (a reduction of at least 50% of urge incontinence episodes) versus 0% in the placebo group. They also noted a statistically significant improvement in number of incontinence episodes, number of voids, voided volume and incontinence quality of life (I-QoL) scores in the PTNS group; none of which was significantly improved in the placebo group.[26]

PTNS is described as well tolerated in both meta-analyses and no serious adverse events were reported.[22,23] Infrequent temporary side effects included pain, bruising, tingling, or bleeding at insertion site, and leg cramp and numbness/pain under the sole of the foot. A study by MacDiarmid and colleagues[27,28] followed PTNS for 6 and 12 months after completing the initial 12 sessions of PTNS to evaluate the long-term efficacy of the intervention. Overactive bladder questionnaire symptom severity was significantly improved from 12 weeks to 12 months (p 0.01) as well as from 6 to 12 months (p 0.01). Overall, current literature on PTNS shows that it is a safe, effective procedure for treatment of symptoms of OAB and effects have been shown to persist up to a year but more long-term data are needed.

Sacral Neuromodulation

Sacral neuromodulation is a method for treating overactive bladder symptoms that are refractory to other methods. Theoretically, sacral neuromodulation is thought to act by activation of afferent sacral nerve fibers that inhibit parasympathetic motor neurons, thereby preventing detrusor contractions. The procedure is often 2-staged, where first an electrode is placed through a sacral foramen to lie close to a sacral nerve, typically S3. The patient undergoes a test phase as a set of programmed electrical impulses are delivered to the electrode within a set range. If the patient has adequate response to the stimulation (reduction in number of voids and episodes of incontinence), then the patient will undergo the second stage of the procedure. Approximately 30% of patients receive little or no response during this phase and do not go on to have the second phase implanted. Phase 2 involves connecting the electrode via cable under the skin to the implantable impulse generator. The procedure requires the operating room and can be costly.

Studies by both van Kerrebroeck and colleagues[29] and Groen and colleagues[30] followed patients being treated for OAB with sacral neuromodulation over time and also monitored for adverse events. Van Kerrebroeck and colleagues[29] collected data from 17 centers and followed 153 patients who had sacral neuromodulation with voiding diaries for 5 years. They reported statistically significant decreases in number of incontinence episodes per day (9.6 ± 6.0 decreased to 3.9 ± 4.0) and number of voids per day (19.3 ± 7.0 decreased to 14.8 ± 7.6). This study reported no life-threatening or irreversible adverse events over 5 years. They defined "success" as a 50% improvement from baseline and reported success rates of 68% for incontinence and 56% for urinary frequency. Groen and colleagues[30] similarly followed patients for 5 years and defined "success" as a 50% decrease in incontinence episodes or pads used daily. At 1 month, 87% of patients reported success and this decreased to 62% by 5 years. They reported 57 adverse events over 5 years but none of the events were severe, per the Clavien grading system.

A literature review by Siddiqui and colleagues[31] published in 2010 sought to review available research regarding the efficacy, particularly with the development of new tined leads, as well as the safety, of sacral neuromodulation devices (specifically Inter-stim [Minneapolis, MN, USA]). Seven studies were of sufficiently good quality to be included in this review of sacral neuromodulation efficacy. In these studies, incontinent episodes per day and pad usage significantly improved after sacral nerve stimulation. Six studies were designated as "good" for review of adverse events. With the new use of tined leads, surgical revision rates ranged from 3% to 16%, which is a decrease from the nontined leads. Six percent of patients had their stimulator removed due to lack of efficacy and 5% to 11% of Interstim devices were explanted due to infection. Overall, the group concluded that sacral nerve stimulation "appears effective for the treatment of overactive bladder in women and adverse event rates with tined leads are lower than previously published estimates using nontined leads."[31] Additional high-quality research with randomized trials is needed to determine the overall efficacy, particularly in comparison with other available treatments, and cost-effectiveness of sacral neuromodulation for long-term treatment of overactive bladder.

SUMMARY

Overactive bladder negatively impacts the quality of life for a large number of patients and is a large economic burden due to necessary costs of health care provider visits, use of pads and other incontinence supplies, medications, and surgical procedures. Along with behavioral modifications, anticholinergics have long been the mainstay of treatment, and the extended-release versions are typically more effective and better tolerated than immediate-release formulations. However, these medications are frequently discontinued over time because of side effects and incomplete resolution of symptoms. Emerging β3-adrenergic agonists provide a medication option with a better side-effect profile. Newer treatment options include onabotulinumtoxinA bladder injections, PTNS, and sacral neuromodulation. Each of these alternatives shows promise in initial research, but more long-term evaluation and comparative studies are needed to definitely recommend one method of treatment over another and to determine which patient would most benefit from each treatment option.

REFERENCES

1. Stewart W, Herzog R, Wein A, et al. The prevalence and impact of overactive bladder in the US: results from the NOBLE program. Neurourol Urodyn 2001; 20:406–8.
2. Onukwugha E, Zuckerman IH, McNally D, et al. The total economic burden of overactive bladder in the United States: a disease-specific approach. Am J Manag Care 2009;15:S90–7.
3. Hu TW, Wagner TH, Bentkover JD, et al. Costs of urinary incontinence and overactive bladder in the United States: a comparative study. Urology 2004;63(3): 461–5.
4. Abrams P, Cardozo L, Fall M, et al. The Standardization of Terminology of Lower Urinary Tract Function: Report from the Standardisation Sub-committee of the International Continence Society. Neurology and Urodynamics 2002;21:167–78.
5. Gormley EA, Lightner DJ, Faraday M, et al. Diagnosis and treatment of overactive bladder (non-neurogenic) in adults: AUA/SUFU guideline. J Urol 2015;193(5): 1572–80.
6. Dumoulin C, Hay-Smith EJC, Mac Habeée-Séguin G. Pelvic floor muscle training versus no treatment, or inactive control treatments, for urinary incontinence in women. Cochrane Database Syst Rev 2014;(5):CD005654.
7. Lucas MG, Bedretdinova D, Bosch JLHR, et al. Guidelines on urinary incontinence. Eur Assoc Urol 2014.

8. Shamliyan T, Wyman J, Kane RL. Nonsurgical treatments for urinary incontinence in adult women: diagnosis and comparative effectiveness. Comparative effectiveness review No. 36. AHRQ Publication No. 11(12)-EHC074-EF. Rockville (MD): Agency for Healthcare Research and Quality; 2012.

9. Madhuvrata P, Cody JD, Ellis G, et al. Which anticholinergic drug for overactive bladder symptoms in adults. Cochrane Database Syst Rev 2012;(1):CD005429.

10. Nabi G, Cody JD, Ellis G, et al. Anticholinergic drugs versus placebo for overactive bladder syndrome in adults. Cochrane Database Syst Rev 2006;(4):CD003781.

11. Kleeman S, Karram M. Overactive bladder syndrome and nocturia. In: Walters M, Karram M, editors. Urogynecology and reconstructive pelvic surgery. 3rd edition. Philadelphia: Mosby Elsevier; 2007. p. 353–76.

12. Fantl JA, Wyman JF, McClish DK, et al. Efficacy of bladder training in older women with urinary incontinence. JAMA 1991;265(5):609–13.

13. Jarvis GJ, Millar DR. Controlled trial of bladder drill for detrusor instability. Br Med J 1980;281(6251):1322–3.

14. Kelleher CJ, Cardozo LD, Khullar V, et al. A medium term analysis of the subjective efficacy of treatment for women with detrusor instability and low bladder compliance. Br J Obs Gynecol 1997;104:988–93.

15. Nitti VW, Dmochowski R, Herschorn S, et al, EMBARK Study Group. OnabotulinumtoxinA for the treatment of patients with overactive bladder and urinary incontinence: results of a phase 3, randomized, placebo controlled trial. J Urol 2013; 189:2186–93.

16. Duthie JB, Vincent M, Herbison GP, et al. Botulinum toxin injections for adults with overactive bladder syndrome. Cochrane Database Syst Rev 2011;(12):CD005493.

17. Visco AG, Brubaker L, Richter HE, et al. Anticholinergic therapy vs. onabotulinumtoxinA for urgency urinary incontinence. Pelvic Floor Disorders Network. N Engl J Med 2012;367:1803–13.

18. Yokoyama T, Chancellor MB, Oguma K, et al. Botulinum toxin type A for the treatment of lower urinary tract disorders. Int J Urol 2012;19:202–15.

19. Popat R, Apostolidis A, Kalsi V, et al. A comparison between the response of patients with idiopathic detrusor overactivity and neurogenic detrusor overactivity to the first intradetrusor injection of botulinum-A toxin. J Urol 2005;174:984–9.

20. Schmid DM, Sauermann P, Werger M, et al. Experience with 100 cases treated with botulinum-A toxin injections in the detrusor muscle for idiopathic overactive bladder syndrome refractory to anticholinergics. J Urol 2006;176:177–85.

21. Compérat E, Reitz A, Delcourt A, et al. Histologic features in the urinary bladder wall affected from neurogenic overactivity–a comparison of inflammation, oedema and fibrosis with and without injection of botulinum toxin type A. Eur Urol 2006;50:1058–64.

22. Gaziev G, Topazio L, Iacovelli V, et al. Percutaneous tibial nerve stimulation (PTNS) efficacy in the treatment of lower urinary tract dysfunctions: a systematic review. BMC Urol 2013;13:61.

23. Burton C, Sajja A, Latthe PM. Effectiveness of percutaneous posterior tibial nerve stimulation for overactive bladder: a systematic review and meta-analysis. Neurourol Urodyn 2012;31:1206–16.

24. Peters KM, Carrico DJ, Perez-Marrero RA, et al. Randomized trial of percutaneous tibial nerve stimulation versus sham efficacy in the treatment of overactive bladder syndrome: results from the SUmiT trial. J Urol 2010;183(4): 1438–43.

25. Peters KM, MacDiarmid SA, Wooldridge LS, et al. Randomized trial of percutaneous tibial nerve stimulation versus extended-release tolterodine: results from the overactive bladder innovative therapy trial. J Urol 2009;182(3):1055–61.

26. Finazzi-Agro E, Petta F, Sciobica F, et al. Percutaneous Tibial Nerve Stimulation effects on detrusor overactivity incontinence are not due to a placebo effect: a randomized double-blind placebo-controlled trial. J Urol 2010;184(5):2001–6.

27. MacDiarmid SA, Peters KM, Shobeiri SA, et al. Long-term durability of percutaneous tibial nerve stimulation for the treatment of overactive bladder. J Urol 2010;183:234–40.

28. Herbison GP, Arnold EP. Sacral neuromodulation with implanted devices for urinary storage and voiding dysfunction in adults. Cochrane Database Syst Rev 2009;(2):CD004202.

29. van Kerrebroeck PE, van Voskuilen AC, Heesakkers JP, Lycklama á Nijholt AA. Results of sacral neuromodulation therapy for urinary voiding dysfunction: outcomes of a prospective, worldwide clinical study. J Urol 2007;178:2029–34.

30. Groen J, Blok BF, Bosch JL. Sacral neuromodulation as treatment for refractory idiopathic urge urinary incontinence: 5-year results of a longitudinal study in 60 women. J Urol 2011;186:954–9.

31. Siddiqui NY, Wu JM, Amundsen CL. Efficacy and adverse events of sacral nerve stimulation for overactive bladder: a systematic review. Neurourol Urodyn 2010; 29(Suppl 1):S18–23.

Native Tissue Prolapse Repairs

Comparative Effectiveness Trials

Lauren N. Siff, MD*, Matthew D. Barber, MD, MHS

KEYWORDS

- Pelvic organ prolapse • Colpopexy • Anterior colporrhaphy • Posterior colporrhaphy
- Uterosacral ligament suspension • Sacrospinous ligament fixation
- Native-tissue pelvic organ prolapse repair • Vaginal reconstruction

KEY POINTS

- Overall, success rates for native tissue prolapse repairs vary widely depending on definition of success used, but generally, risk of prolapse beyond the hymen is 10% to 15%, recurrent vaginal bulging symptoms are 10% to 20%, and need for reoperation is less than 10% 1 to 2 years after surgery.
- Uterosacral ligament suspension and sacrospinous ligament fixation are equally as effective in the treatment of apical pelvic organ prolapse at 2 years postoperatively.
- Ultralateral suturing and standard midline plication are equally as effective in treatment of anterior pelvic organ prolapse; the addition of absorbable mesh graft does not improve outcomes.
- Transvaginal approach to rectocele repair is superior to transanal approach.
- Midline plication is as effective as site-specific repair in treatment of symptomatic rectocele, and addition of a porcine-derived biologic graft provides inferior results in the posterior compartment.

INTRODUCTION

The lifetime risk of undergoing at least one surgical procedure for pelvic organ prolapse (POP) ranges from 6%[1] to 19%.[2] Retrospective 5-year follow-up data after approximately 700 vaginal native-tissue POP repairs by Oversand and colleagues[3] showed reoperation rates of 2.6% to 8.9% and final conclusions that native tissue POP surgery "should be the first choice in treating primary POP." The 2013 Cochrane Review of surgical management of POP highlights the risks and benefits when

Center for Urogynecology and Reconstructive Pelvic Surgery, Obstetrics, Gynecology & Women's Health Institute, Cleveland Clinic, 9500 Euclid Avenue A81, Cleveland, OH 44195, USA
* Corresponding author. 9500 Euclid Avenue, A81, Cleveland Clinic, Cleveland, OH 44195.
E-mail address: siffl@ccf.org

Obstet Gynecol Clin N Am 43 (2016) 69–81
http://dx.doi.org/10.1016/j.ogc.2015.10.003
obgyn.theclinics.com
0889-8545/16/$ – see front matter © 2016 Elsevier Inc. All rights reserved.

choosing appropriate surgical approach to POP repairs particularly, in comparing native tissue repairs to graft-augmented repair of all compartments. The benefit of graft augmentation versus native tissue repair clearly varies from the apex to the anterior and posterior compartments; however, the recurring theme in all compartments is to balance improved surgical outcomes against longer operating time, increased blood loss, longer time to return to activities of daily living, increased cost, and reoperation rate for mesh exposures associated with graft augmentation.[4] This article reviews the success rates and complications of native tissue vaginal reconstruction procedures for pelvic organ prolapse from randomized clinical trials and other comparative studies by compartment (the vaginal apex, anterior and posterior compartments). Trials comparing native tissue repair with synthetic mesh augmented repairs (sacrocolpopexy and vaginal mesh) can be found in chapter entitle "Pelvic Organ Prolapse— Vaginal and Laparoscopic Mesh: The Evidence" by Sokol and colleagues.[5]

DEFINING SUCCESS OF SURGERY FOR PELVIC ORGAN PROLAPSE

Success rates after prolapse surgeries vary widely depending on the definition used. When strict anatomic criteria are used (pelvic organ prolapse quantification [POP-Q] stage 0 or 1), success rates of native tissue prolapse repair are generally low (37%–64% in several trials).[6–8] However, 30% to 65% of women who receive routine gynecologic care without prolapse symptoms have POP-Q stage 2 vaginal support on straining examination, and 3% to 6% even have prolapse beyond the hymen. Therefore, strict anatomic criteria do not seem appropriate, as a substantial proportion of women in the general population without symptoms of POP would not meet these criteria. When more clinically relevant criteria are used, such as no prolapse beyond the hymen, anatomic success rates are considerably better (82%–94%).

To further illustrate this point, Barber and colleagues[9] tested 18 permutations to define surgical success and used these to reanalyze the data of the Colpopexy and Urinary Reduction Efforts (CARE) trial. These definitions used POP-Q assessments, responses to Pelvic Floor Distress Inventory questions regarding vaginal bulging, data on retreatment (surgery or pessary), and participants' subjective ratings of overall treatment success and global improvement. Recommendations for developing the most clinically relevant definition for surgical success were based on showing a significantly better global impression of improvement, lower symptom bother (lower Pelvic Floor Distress Inventory scores), and higher health-related quality of life (lower Pelvic Floor Impact Questionnaire scores) in treatment successes than in failures. They found that the absence of vaginal bulge symptoms postoperatively has a significant relationship with a patient's assessment of overall improvement and improvement in quality of life after surgery, whereas anatomic success alone does not.[9] Perhaps the most clinically relevant criteria for success, particularly for the patient, are symptomatic cure, specifically absence of vaginal bulge symptoms.[9,10] Subjective cure after native tissue pelvic organ prolapse repairs is high (82%–96%) in those studies in which it has been reported. Similarly, reoperations for recurrent prolapse in almost all trials are less than 10% with most at ≤5%.

When interpreting the results of trials comparing surgical efficacy, it becomes important to keep in mind the varying definitions of success and those that are most clinically meaningful. Good outcome measures are essential to compare one treatment with another, to compare our own results with those of another, and perhaps, most importantly, to counsel our patients effectively, realistically, and honestly using outcomes that are relevant to the individual patient.[9] In designing future studies, the definition of success after POP surgery should include the absence of bulge symptoms and the absence of retreatment in addition to anatomic criteria. Using the hymen as a threshold for anatomic success seems most appropriate.[9,10] As these outcome measures are being adopted, we can more accurately compare one treatment with another.

VAGINAL APEX

Native tissue prolapse repairs to restore the vaginal apex include McCall's culdoplasty, iliococcygeus fixation (ICS), sacrospinous ligament fixation (SSLF) (**Fig. 1**), and uterosacral ligament suspension (USLS) (**Fig. 2**). Data describing McCall's culdoplasty and ICS for treatment of pelvic organ prolapse are limited to observational study designs.[11–13] Maher and colleagues[11] in 2001 performed a retrospective case-control study comparing ICS (n = 50) with SSLF (n = 78). Subjective and objective successes were similar between the 2 groups (91 vs 94% and 54 vs 67%, respectively). Serati and colleagues[12] reported surgical success rates of ICS on 44 women after a median follow-up of 69 months. The composite success rates, including both subjective and objective measures and reoperation, were 84.1% (37 of 44). Only preoperative stage IV vaginal vault prolapse independently predicted POP recurrence after ICS (odds ratio [OR], 8.78; 95% confidence interval [CI], 1.31–9.42]; $P<.001$).

Currently, data regarding McCall's culdoplasty are limited to retrospective series with reoperation rates for POP ranging from 0% to 14%.[14]

The Comparison of 2 Transvaginal Surgical Approaches and Perioperative Behavioral Therapy for Apical Vaginal Prolapse (The OPTIMAL Trial)[15] is the largest prospective clinical trial of 2 native tissue surgical approaches to the repair of apical POP. OPTIMAL is a multicenter (9 US medical centers), multisurgeon, 2 × 2 factorial randomized trial of 374 women undergoing surgery to treat apical vaginal prolapse and stress urinary incontinence. Patients were followed up closely for 2 years with rate

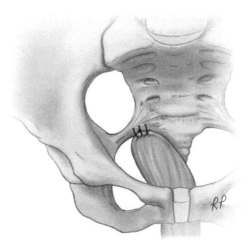

Fig. 1. Sacrospinous ligament fixation. (*Courtesy of* Cleveland Clinic Center for Medical Art & Photography, ©2012–2015; with permission.)

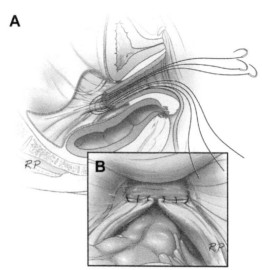

Fig. 2. Uterosacral ligament suspension. (*Courtesy of* Cleveland Clinic Center for Medical Art & Photography, ©2012–2015; with permission.)

of follow-up of 84.5%. The primary outcome for surgical intervention was composite surgical success defined as (1) no apical descent greater than 1/3 into the vaginal canal or anterior or posterior vaginal wall beyond the hymen, (2) no bothersome vaginal bulge symptoms, and (3) no retreatment for prolapse at 24 months. The primary outcome for the behavioral intervention was measured by (1) urinary symptoms scores (urinary distress inventory range, 0–300) at 6 months, (2) prolapse symptoms scores (pelvic organ prolapse distress inventory range, 0–300) at 24 months, and (3) anatomic success (as defined above) at 24 months. There were no clinically significant differences in any of the primary outcome components between groups. Surgical success was not different between the USLS versus SSLF groups with rates of 64.5% (100 of 155) versus 63.1% (94 of 149) (adjusted OR, 1.1; 95% CI, 0.7–1.7). An illustration representation of SSLF and USLS are seen in **Figs. 1** and **2**. Overall, 18% of women (55 of 305) had bothersome vaginal bulge symptoms, 14.6% (45 of 308) had anterior or posterior or both beyond the hymen, and 5.1% (16 of 316) underwent retreatment either with a pessary or surgery.

Participants randomly assigned to the perioperative behavioral therapy with pelvic floor muscle training (BPMT) group received an individualized program that included 1 visit 2 to 4 weeks before surgery and 4 postoperative visits (2, 4–6, 8, and 12 weeks after surgery). Pelvic floor muscle training, individualized progressive pelvic floor muscle exercise, and education on behavioral strategies to reduce urinary and colorectal symptoms were performed at each visit. Usual perioperative care included routine perioperative teaching and standardized postoperative instructions. There were no significant differences in the BPMT, and usual care for 6- and 24- month primary outcomes (composite success). The anterior vagina was the most likely compartment to prolapse beyond the hymen (not different between BPMT vs usual care; 12.1% vs 13.8%) In women receiving usual care, those in USLS were less likely to have apical descent than those with SSLF (4.9% vs 15.6%; adjusted OR, 0.3; 95% CI, 0.1–0.8). In women receiving BMPT, there was no difference in apical descent (USLS 16.2% vs SSLF 12.0%; adjusted OR, 1.4;

95% CI, 0.6–3.7). Women in the SSLF group were no more likely to have recurrence with or without BPMT.

Both USLS and SSLF are safe procedures with less than 5% of serious adverse events over a 2-year follow-up period that were directly related to the index surgery. In terms of adverse events, ureteral obstruction was seen in 3.7% (3.2% [n = 5] was diagnosed intraoperatively and 0.5% [n = 1] was diagnosed postoperatively). All of the ureteral obstructions were in the USLS group, and none were identified in the SSLF group. The rate of acute neurologic pain (namely buttock pain), possibly as a result of gluteal nerve entrapment, was 4.3% with persistent pain beyond 6 weeks. All of these patients belonged to the SSLF group; there was no acute neurologic pain in the USLS group.

The conclusions of the OPTIMAL Trial were that 2 years after vaginal surgery for prolapse and stress urinary incontinence, neither USLS nor SSLF were superior to the other for anatomic, function, or adverse event outcomes. Perioperative BPMT did not improve prolapse outcomes at 2 years.

ANTERIOR COMPARTMENT

One randomized, masked trial compares anterior vaginal prolapse native tissue repairs with one another. Weber and colleagues[6] performed a prospective, randomized trial including 114 patients who were randomly assigned to standard anterior colporrhaphy with midline plication, ultralateral native tissue colporrhaphy with dissection taken laterally to the limits of the pubic rami, or standard colporrhaphy plus polyglactin mesh graft placement. The primary outcome measured was anatomic success (with optimal cure being stage 0, and satisfactory cure being stage I anterior wall prolapse). Failure was defined as stage II or greater (Aa, Ba ≤-1). An independent observer performed follow-up examinations and compared postoperative and preoperative symptom questionnaires at 6, 12, and 24 months after surgery. The cure rate in this study was 38% by strict anatomic criteria with median follow-up of 23 months. Most patients had anatomic results at the level of the hymen with relatively low rates of elevation above stage 2. There was, however, a high rate of symptomatic improvement with a mean change in visual analog scales seen for prolapse symptoms of 5.7 ± 2.8 points, urinary symptoms of 2.5 ± 3.9 points, and sexual function of 2.4 ± 3.9 points. Based on this study, there does not seem to be an advantage of one suturing technique over another for anterior colporrhaphy in terms of anatomic or symptomatic result. The addition of absorbable mesh to traditional repair did not substantially improve cure rates.

Chmielewski and colleagues[16] reanalyzed the data from the Weber trial using definition of success as (1) no prolapse beyond the hymen, (2) no bothersome bulge symptoms, and (3) no retreatment (with repeat surgery or a pessary). With this updated definition of success, at 1 year after surgery, success of anterior repair was 88% with no differences between standard colporrhaphy, ultralateral suturing, or absorbable mesh-augment repair. This finding illustrates that surgical outcomes can vary greatly based on the definition of success. A 38% rate of strict anatomic success 2 years after surgery may be unacceptably low to continue offering native tissue anterior repair as treatment of anterior vaginal wall prolapse, however; once a more clinically relevant definition of treatment success was applied, the results substantiate native tissue repair.

Somewhat contradictory to the results of Weber's trial, Sand and colleagues[7] randomly assigned 160 women with anterior vaginal wall prolapse beyond the hymen who were planning to undergo pelvic reconstructive surgery to receive or not to receive polyglactin 910 absorbable mesh at the time of anterior colporrhaphy. For patients who received the polyglactin mesh, one piece of mesh was imbricated into the endopelvic connective tissue beneath the trigone, and a second piece was imbricated into the endopelvic connective tissue just anterior to the vaginal cuff (a third piece of mesh was used in the posterior compartment if patient was undergoing rectocele repair). The addition of mesh added only seconds to the procedure. Patients in each group were compared at baseline, 12 weeks, and 1 year after surgery. Primary outcomes were recurrent cystocele to the midvaginal plane or beyond. Central cystocele recurred in 22% (16 of 73) women in the mesh group and 40% (28 of 70) in the nonmesh group (P = .02). When considering recurrent anterior wall prolapse beyond the hymen, only 1 of 73 in the mesh group and 8 of 70 in the no-mesh group had recurrence (P = .01). Suburethral sling placement was found to be associated with a significantly lower risk of recurrent cystocele, but the independent effect of mesh placement on the anterior vaginal wall recurrence remained statistically significant after control for suburethral sling placement (OR, 0.48; 95% CI, 0.23–1.00; P = .05). There was no effect of this mesh on the success of posterior colporrhaphy.

POSTERIOR COMPARTMENT

Three randomized trials are available that compare suturing technique and surgical approach with native tissue posterior vaginal wall prolapse repair. The first trial by Paraiso and colleagues[17] sought to compare anatomic and functional outcomes of 3 surgical techniques for rectocele repair: (1) posterior colporrhaphy, (2) site-specific repair, and (3) porcine-derived, graft-augmented, site-specific repair. Posterior colporrhaphies were performed as a midline plication using ethibond, and no levator plication was done. Graft augmented repairs attached the graft to the levator ani fascia laterally, the vault suspension (if performed) superiorly, and the perineal body inferiorly. Perineorrhaphy was performed if the patient reported splinting to defecate or a perineal defect noted on examination. Patients included in this trial had stage 2 or greater posterior vaginal wall prolapse and desired surgical repair. The primary outcome was anatomic cure defined as POP-Q point Bp $\leq$-1 one year after surgery. Functional outcomes were defined by worsening of the prolapse (POPDI-6) and colorectal (CRADI-8) specific sections of the pelvic floor distress inventory (PFDI-20).[18] Dyspareunia was defined as an affirmative response to the PISQ-12 question "do you feel pain during sexual intercourse," and defecatory dysfunction was defined as the need to strain, splint, or incomplete emptying with defecation.

One year after surgery, anatomic cure rates between the standard colporrhaphy (86%) and site-specific repair (78%) were significantly greater than those with graft augmentation (54%; P = .02). Twenty percent of graft-augmented repairs had prolapse beyond the hymen at 1 year compared with 7.1% standard colporrhaphy and 7.4% site-specific repair (P = .27). Reoperation rate was 3% in standard colporrhaphy, 5% in site-specific repair, and 10% in graft-augmented repair. All participants had functional outcome improvement with surgery, and no difference was seen among groups; however a proportion of each group had worsening colorectal and prolapse symptoms 1 year postoperatively (16% standard colporrhaphy, 12% of site specific, 21% graft augmented); however, these changes did not reach statistical significance. Defecatory dysfunction and sexual function improved in all patients with no difference among groups. Dyspareunia was present in 20% standard colporrhaphy, 14% site-specific repair, and 6% graft-augmented repair

1 year after surgery with no difference among groups. Overall, 93% of subjects indicated they would choose the same treatment again with no difference among groups. The conclusions of this trial show that posterior colporrhaphy and site-specific rectocele repair result in similar anatomic and functional outcomes. The addition of porcine-derived graft does not improve anatomic outcomes, and all 3 methods of rectocele repair result in significant improvements in symptoms, quality of life (QOL) and sexual function.

Sung and colleagues[19] somewhat contradict the above findings from Paraiso and colleagues in that they do not see inferior outcomes with use of a porcine-derived graft versus native issue for rectocele repair, perhaps because a different graft was used. However, they did find that porcine subintestinal submucosal graft augmentation was not superior to native tissue for anatomic or subjective outcomes 12 months after rectocele repair. They randomly assigned 160 women with stage 2 or greater symptomatic rectoceles from 2 sites to receive rectocele repair with or without porcine graft. Both the graft and no-graft group were allowed to receive midline plication or site-specific repair based on surgeon preference, and no levator plications were performed. Subjective failure was defined as no improvement or worsening of symptoms, anatomic failure was defined as points Ap or Bp -1 or greater on blinded POP-Q. There was no difference between graft (n = 67) versus No-graft (n = 70) groups in anatomic failure (12% vs 9%; $P = .5$), vaginal bulge symptom failure (3% vs 7%; $P = .4$), or defecatory symptom failure (44% vs 45%; $P = .9$).

The second trial comparing effectiveness of surgical approach in the native tissue repair of posterior vaginal wall prolapse is authored by Nieminen and colleagues.[20] This is a randomized trial comparing transanal versus transvaginal approach to rectocele repair. Thirty women with symptomatic rectoceles underwent either transanal rectoceleplasty (n = 15) or posterior colporrhaphy (n = 15). The patients were assessed by physical examination, defecography, and anorectal manometry at baseline and 12 months postoperatively. Patients were excluded if they had disrupted anal sphincter function or other symptomatic pelvic organ prolapse.

Preoperatively, 73% (11 of 15) in the transvaginal group and 66% (10 of 15) in the transanal group splinted to defecate. One year after surgery, 93% (14 of 15) in the transvaginal group and 73% (11 of 15) in transanal group reported improvement in symptoms; only 1 (7%) in the transvaginal and 4 (27%) in transanal had to splint postoperatively. Recurrence rates were 7% (1 of 15) versus 40% (6 of 15) in transvaginal versus transanal groups. Patient's symptoms were significantly alleviated by both techniques, but the transanal technique was associated with more clinically diagnosed recurrences. None of the patients reported de novo dyspareunia, and 27% reported improvement.

The third prospective 3-arm randomized trial regarding to rectocele repair is by Farid and colleagues[21] The investigators randomly assigned patients to transperineal versus transanal repairs of rectoceles associated with obstructed defecation. Multiparous women with rectoceles greater than 2 cm and one or more of the following symptoms—a need to splint, a sense of incomplete evacuation, excessive straining, or dyspareunia—were randomly assigned to one of 3 rectocele repairs: (1) transperineal repair with levatorplasty, (2) transperineal repair without levatorplasty, or (3) transanal repair. They then had defecography, anal manometry, physical examinations, and questionnaires measured at baseline and 6 months. Their outcome measures were size of rectocele on defecography, emptying of rectocele, symptomatic improvement, and postoperative sexual function.

At 6 months, preoperative symptoms including sense of incomplete emptying, and straining were statistically significantly improved only in the 2 transperineal groups (not the transanal group). Significant reduction in mean anal resting pressure, maximum reflex volume, and urge-to-defecate volume were observed with both transperineal approaches (not transanal group). Levatorplasty significantly improved the overall functional score compared with transperineal repair alone but increased the incidence of dyspareunia. This trial concluded that rectocele repair improves ano-rectal function by improving rectal urge sensitivity. Transperineal repair is superior to transanal repair in structural and functional outcomes. Levatorplasty improves functional outcome but increases the rates of dyspareunia and should be avoided in sexually active women.

UTERINE PRESERVATION

The ideas that the uterus is an innocent bystander in a poorly supported vagina and that hysterectomy is not necessarily required for pelvic organ prolapse repair are being presented more and more. Some patients, for personal reasons, prefer a uterine-sparing procedure. In the recent review by Ridgeway,[22] "uterine-sparing procedures require more research but remain an acceptable option for most patients with utero-vaginal prolapse after a balanced and unbiased discussion reviewing the advantages and disadvantages of this approach."

Currently, 2 published prospective randomized trials compare hysteropexy with total vaginal hysterectomy (TVH) with native tissue reconstruction. The first trial by Dietz and colleagues[23] is a multicenter multisurgeon randomized, controlled trial that randomly assigned 66 women with stage 2 to 4 uterovaginal prolapse to TVH with USLS or sacrospinous hysteropexy (SSH). Both procedures included anterior colporrhaphy, posterior colporrhaphy, or both. Outcomes included recovery time, anatomic outcome, functional outcomes, and QOL. The primary outcome, return to work, was shorter after SSH (43 vs 66 days; $P = .02$). Recurrent stage 2 or greater apical prolapse 1 year postoperatively was 27% in the SSH group (with a reoperation rate of 11% [4 of 35]) versus 3% apical recurrence in the TVH group (reoperation rate [anterior/posterior colporrhaphies] of 7% [2 of 31]). There were no differences in QOL 1 year postoperatively. Complications were rare, but one ureteral obstruction was noted in the TVH group (none in the SSH group). The conclusions of this trial show that SSH for uterine descent is associated with earlier recovery time, more recurrent prolapsed, and no difference in functional outcome or QOL.

The second trial by Detollenaere and colleagues[24] sought to investigate whether uterus-preserving vaginal sacrospinous hysteropexy is noninferior to vaginal hysterectomy with suspension of the uterosacral ligaments in the surgical treatment of uterine prolapse. This is a multicenter, randomized, noninferiority trial comparing 208 women with stage 2 or greater uterine prolapse who desire surgical management and have no history of prior pelvic floor surgery. Concomitant anterior and posterior repairs were allowed as well as anti-incontinence procedures as desired by the surgeon. The primary outcome was composite surgical success including no evidence of recurrent stage 2 or greater apical prolapse, bothersome bulge symptoms, and no retreatment (surgery or pessary) 12 months after surgery. Secondary outcomes were stage 2 or greater recurrent prolapse in any compartment (including anterior and posterior) with bothersome bulge symptoms and retreatment for recurrent prolapse of any compartment. Data regarding functional outcomes, complications, hospital stay, postoperative recovery, and sexual function were collected at baseline, 6 weeks, 6 months, and 12 months and continued annually for 60 months. The SSH was performed via a posterior approach to the sacrospinous ligament followed by placement of 2 permanent sutures through the ligament at least 2 cm medial to the ischial spine. Patients underwent preoperative pap smear and pelvic ultrasound scan to evaluate for uterine or cervical conditions before surgery.

The primary outcome of this trial was recurrent apical prolapse, bothersome bulge symptoms, or retreatment. With this definition, the composite surgical failure rate in SSH group was 0%, and TVH USLS was 4%. When looking at anatomic outcomes of any compartment stage 2 or greater, it was 50% in the SSH and 44% in the TVH USLS groups. Fifty-one of 101 patients in the SSH had recurrences, and 44 of 100 in the TVH USLS group had recurrences. These were mostly anterior wall recurrences (47 of 101 SSH versus 33 of 99 TVH) with no difference between procedure groups. In the posterior compartment, there was a significantly higher rate of recurrence in TVH USLS group with 14% (14 of 99) versus 4% (4 of 101) in SSH group. Nine patients in SSH group reported buttock pain, but 8 of the 9 experienced symptom resolution by 6 weeks after surgery. Operating time in the SSH group was shorter than that in the TVH USLS group (59±13 minutes vs 72±21 minutes; the difference in the SSH vs TVH USLS was -13.5 (95% CI [-18.5,-8.6]).

The conclusion of this trial was that SSH is noninferior to TVH with USLS for composite surgical success in management of apical uterovaginal prolapse. Overall anatomic outcome, functional outcome, hospital stay, complications, postoperative recovery, and sexual function did not differ between procedures.

DISCUSSION

There is high-quality evidence to support the use of native tissue reconstructive repairs as surgical treatment of bothersome symptomatic prolapse of all compartments (**Table 1**). When clinically relevant definitions of success are used, these repairs have high rates of success (both subjective and objective), low rates of reoperation, and low rates of adverse events. For apical prolapse, both USLSs and SSLFs are effective and provided similar outcomes in anatomy and function with few adverse events. Approximately 18% of women will have bothersome vaginal bulge symptoms, 15% will have anterior or posterior or both beyond the hymen, and 5% will undergo retreatment either with a pessary or surgery 2 years after surgery. Transient ureteral obstruction (4%) was an adverse event specific to USLS, and buttock pain (4%) was specific to SSLF. In the anterior compartment traditional colporrhaphy, the technique is no different than that of ultralateral suturing with anatomic success rates of 38% at 2 years postoperatively; the addition of mesh augmentation does not substantially increase cure rates. In the posterior compartment, transvaginal rectocele repair is superior to transanal repair. Both standard midline plication and site-specific repairs are equally as successful in repairing a symptomatic rectocele (success rates 86% vs 78% at 1 year). The addition of biologic graft to site-specific rectocele repair provides inferior rates of success (54%). For uterine preservation, sacrospinous hysteropexy is not inferior to vaginal hysterectomy with USLS for treatment of apical uterovaginal prolapse. The recurrence of stage 2 or greater POP in any compartment is 50% (SSH) versus 44% (TVH USLS) 1 year postoperatively. SSH is associated with decreased operating time and earlier recovery but increased buttock pain compared with TVH USLS. The data provided in this review of comparative effectiveness trials can aid in patient counseling and procedure selection when surgically treating patients with native tissue vaginal reconstruction POP repairs.

Table 1
Comparative trials of native tissue pelvic organ prolapse repairs

Study/Design	Procedure (n)	Mean Follow-up	Anatomic Success	Subjective Success (%)	Retreatment Rate (%)	Complications	Comments/Conclusion
Apex							
Maher et al,[11] 2001/ Case-Control	ICS vs SSLF (n = 138)	21 vs 19 mo	(<BW grade 2) 54% vs 67%	91 vs 94	3 vs 0	Transfusion (3% vs 3%) Buttock pain (19% vs 24%)	SSLF = ICS for VVP
Serati et al,[12] 2015/ Prospective Observational	ICS (n = 44)	69 mo	(<POPQ stage 2) 84%	89	4.5	None	—
Barber et al,[15] 2014/RCT	USLS vs SSLF (n = 374)	24 mo	(<Hymen) 84% vs 86%	83 vs 80	5	Buttock pain >6 wk (0% vs 4%) Ureteral obstruction (3.7% vs 0%)	USLS = SSLF
Anterior Compartment							
Weber et al,[6] 2001/ RCT	AR (n = 114) Standard repair Ultralateral repair Graft-augmented repair	23 mo	(<POPQ stage 2) 30% 46% 42%	n/r	n/r	None	No difference in anatomic cure rates among groups
Chmielewski et al,[16] 2011/RCT	AR (n = 114)	23 mo	(<Hymen) 82%	94	3	None	—
Sand et al,[7] 2001/ RCT	AR (n = 160) Absorbable mesh No mesh	12 mo	(<Hymen) 98% 89%	n/r	n/r	None	Absorbable mesh > no mesh

Posterior Compartment

			POPQ Bp ≥0				
Paraiso et al,[17] 2006/RCT	PR (n = 105) Standard repair Site-specific repair Porcine graft	18 mo	93% 93% 80%	84 88 79	3 5 10	Transfusion (8% vs 0% vs 3%) Postoperative infection (11% vs 0% v 3%) No graft exposures	Standard repair = site-specific porcine graft is inferior
Sung et al,[19] 2012/ RCT	PR (n = 160) Porcine graft No graft	12 mo	(<POPQ stage 2) 88% 91%	97 93	n/r	n/r No graft exposures	Graft = no graft
Uterine Preservation							
Dietz et al,[23] 2010/ RCT	SSH vs TVH/USLS (n = 66)	12 mo	(Apex < POP-Q stage 2) 73% vs 97%	n/r	11 vs 7	Ureteral obstruction 0% vs 3%	SSH = TVH/USLS
Detollenaere et al,[24] 2015	SSH vs TVH/USLS (n = 208)	12 mo	(Apex < POP-Q stage 2) 100% vs 96%	n/r	2 vs 0	Buttock pain >6 wk 1% vs 0%	SSH is not inferior to TVH/USLS for apical prolapse

Abbreviations: AR, anterior repair; BW, Baden-Walker; n/r, not reported; PR, posterior repair; RCT, randomized controlled trial; VVP, vaginal vault prolapse. *Data from* Refs.[6,7,11,12,15-17,19,23,24]

REFERENCES

1. Olsen AL, Smith VJ, Bergstrom JO, et al. Epidemiology of surgically managed pelvic organ prolapse and urinary incontinence. Obstet Gynecol 1997;89(4): 501–6.
2. Smith FJ, Holman CD, Moorin RE, et al. Lifetime risk of undergoing surgery for pelvic organ prolapse. Obstet Gynecol 2010;116(5):1096–100.
3. Oversand SH, Staff AC, Spydslaug AE, et al. Long-term follow-up after native tissue repair for pelvic organ prolapse. Int Urogynecol J 2014;25(1):81–9.
4. Maher C, Feiner B, Baessler K, et al. Surgical management of pelvic organ prolapse in women. Cochrane Database Syst Rev 2013;(4):CD004014.
5. Richter LA, Sokol AI. Pelvic Organ Prolapse— Vaginal and Laparoscopic Mesh: The Evidence. Obstet Gynecol Clin N Am 2016;43(1):83–92.
6. Weber AM, Walters MD, Piedmonte MR, et al. Anterior colporrhaphy: a randomized trial of three surgical techniques. Am J Obstet Gynecol 2001;185(6): 1299–304 [discussion: 1304–6].
7. Sand PK, Koduri S, Lobel RW, et al. Prospective randomized trial of polyglactin 910 mesh to prevent recurrence of cystoceles and rectoceles. Am J Obstet Gynecol 2001;184(7):1357–62 [discussion: 1362–4].
8. Barber MD, Brubaker L, Menefee S, et al. Operations and pelvic muscle training in the management of apical support loss (OPTIMAL) trial: design and methods. Contemp Clin Trials 2009;30(2):178–89.
9. Barber MD, Brubaker L, Nygaard I, et al. Defining success after surgery for pelvic organ prolapse. Obstet Gynecol 2009;114(3):600–9.
10. Maher C, Baessler K, Barber M, et al. Pelvic organ prolapse surgery. In: Abrams P, Cardozo L, Khoury S, et al, editors. 5th international consultation on incontinence. 5th edition. Paris: Health Publication Ltd; 2013. p. 1377–433.
11. Maher CF, Murray CJ, Carey MP, et al. Iliococcygeus or sacrospinous fixation for vaginal vault prolapse. Obstet Gynecol 2001;98(1):40–4.
12. Serati M, Braga A, Bogani G, et al. Iliococcygeus fixation for the treatment of apical vaginal prolapse: efficacy and safety at 5 years of follow-up. Int Urogynecol J 2015;26(7):1007–12.
13. Milani R, Cesana MC, Spelzini F, et al. Iliococcygeus fixation or abdominal sacral colpopexy for the treatment of vaginal vault prolapse: a retrospective cohort study. Int Urogynecol J 2014;25(2):279–84.
14. Barber MD, Maher C. Apical prolapse. Int Urogynecol J 2013;24(11):1815–33.
15. Barber MD, Brubaker L, Burgio KL, et al. Comparison of 2 transvaginal surgical approaches and perioperative behavioral therapy for apical vaginal prolapse: the OPTIMAL randomized trial. JAMA 2014;311(10):1023–34.
16. Chmielewski L, Walters MD, Weber AM, et al. Reanalysis of a randomized trial of 3 techniques of anterior colporrhaphy using clinically relevant definitions of success. Am J Obstet Gynecol 2011;205(1):69.e1–8.
17. Paraiso MF, Barber MD, Muir TW, et al. Rectocele repair: a randomized trial of three surgical techniques including graft augmentation. Am J Obstet Gynecol 2006;195(6):1762–71.
18. Barber MD, Walters MD, Bump RC. Short forms of two condition-specific quality-of-life questionnaires for women with pelvic floor disorders (PFDI-20 and PFIQ-7). Am J Obstet Gynecol 2005;193(1):103–13.
19. Sung VW, Rardin CR, Raker CA, et al. Porcine subintestinal submucosal graft augmentation for rectocele repair: a randomized controlled trial. Obstet Gynecol 2012;119(1):125–33.

20. Nieminen K, Hiltunen KM, Laitinen J, et al. Transanal or vaginal approach to rectocele repair: a prospective, randomized pilot study. Dis Colon Rectum 2004; 47(10):1636–42.
21. Farid M, Madbouly KM, Hussein A, et al. Randomized controlled trial between perineal and anal repairs of rectocele in obstructed defecation. World J Surg 2010;34(4):822–9.
22. Ridgeway BM. Does prolapse equal hysterectomy? The role of uterine conservation in women with uterovaginal prolapse. Am J Obstet Gynecol 2015. [Epub ahead of print].
23. Dietz V, van der Vaart CH, van der Graaf Y, et al. One-year follow-up after sacrospinous hysteropexy and vaginal hysterectomy for uterine descent: a randomized study. Int Urogynecol J 2010;21(2):209–16.
24. Detollenaere RJ, den Boon J, Stekelenburg J, et al. Sacrospinous hysteropexy versus vaginal hysterectomy with suspension of the uterosacral ligaments in women with uterine prolapse stage 2 or higher: multicentre randomised non-inferiority trial. BMJ 2015;351:h3717.

Pelvic Organ Prolapse— Vaginal and Laparoscopic Mesh: The Evidence

Lee A. Richter, MD*, Andrew I. Sokol, MD

KEYWORDS

- Pelvic organ prolapse • Mesh • Sacrocolpopexy • Laparoscopy • Outcomes

KEY POINTS

- Transvaginal mesh (TVM) repair of the anterior compartment is associated with improved anatomic support compared with native tissue repair, but without significant improvement in quality-of-life parameters.
- Studies fail to show a difference in quality-of-life improvement between vaginal mesh and native tissue vaginal repairs in any compartment.
- Sacral colpopexy is considered the gold standard for management of apical prolapse because of high success rates and few complications.
- Minimally invasive sacrocolpopexy (SCP) has the additional benefit of reduced blood loss and decreased hospital length of stay compared with open SCP, without compromising anatomic or subjective outcomes.
- Level 1 evidence has shown no difference in anatomic or subjective outcomes between the laparoscopic versus robotic SCP.

INTRODUCTION

Approximately 20% of women will undergo surgery for stress urinary incontinence or pelvic organ prolapse (POP) over their lifetime, and a large percentage will require additional surgery for recurrent POP.[1] In an effort to reduce failure rates, graft materials were introduced to augment reconstructive repairs. Based on the success of mesh-augmented repairs for groin hernias, the idea of using synthetic grafts for prolapse repairs developed. The first synthetic mesh prostheses placed abdominally

Disclosures: Dr L.A. Richter is the recipient of a Pfizer Investigator Initiated Grant.
Departments of Obstetrics and Gynecology, and Urology, National Center for Advanced Pelvic Surgery, MedStar Washington Hospital Center, 106 Irving Street NW POB South #405, Washington, DC 20010, USA
* Corresponding author.
E-mail address: Lee.Ann.Richter@medstar.net

for POP repairs were introduced in the 1970s. These synthetic materials, which are fibers woven into mesh form, vary in pore size, filament structure, strength, and inflammatory response. Mesh products that are lightweight, composed of monofilament fibers, and woven into a macroporous architecture are thought to enhance mesh performance because they promote better integration into the host tissue.[2] Currently, the preferred mesh for prolapse repairs is a nonabsorbable synthetic material that meets these characteristics (ie, light-weight, large-pore polypropylene). In this report, current evidence regarding the use of synthetic mesh for the correction of POP is reviewed, and its use in abdominal, laparoscopic, and vaginal surgery is examined.

BACKGROUND ON ABDOMINAL MESH

The sacrocolpopexy (SCP) procedure, generally considered the gold standard surgical procedure for apical POP, was first described in the late 1950s. This procedure, of anchoring the uterus or vaginal apex posteriorly to the sacral promontory, was a novel idea and attempted to reduce the rates of recurrent enterocele that pelvic surgeons had previously encountered when affixing the vagina anteriorly. Use of a graft material was introduced in the early 1960s in order to reduce excessive tension on the apex after elevation.[3] Based on the success of surgical mesh for the repair of abdominal wall hernias, gynecologists began using surgical mesh indicated for hernia repair in their abdominal prolapse repairs in the 1970s. In an attempt to avoid some of the risks associated with synthetic mesh material, surgeons also investigated the use of biologic grafts for the SCP procedure. Of the various types of biologic grafts introduced (porcine dermis, porcine small intestine submucosa, and cadaveric fascia lata), all were shown to be inferior to synthetic mesh for improving apical anatomic support (**Table 1**).[4] In 2001, the US Food and Drug Administration (FDA) officially approved synthetic grafts for use in POP repairs.

The abdominal SCP has robust level 1 evidence to support its success, with proven durability in multiple studies. The long-term follow-up of the randomized

Table 1
Sacral colpopexy outcomes for apical prolapse, biologic grafts compared with synthetic grafts

Author	Graft Type	Number	Follow-up (mo)	Success Rate	Study Design
Cundiff et al, 2008	Pelvicol, Mersilene, Gynemesh, Gore-Tex	302	24	N/A	RCT, secondary analysis
Culligan et al, 2005	Tutoplast, Trelex	89	12	Tutoplast: 68% Trelex: 91%	RCT
Deprest et al, 2009	Xenograft (Surgisis or Pelvicol) vs Gynemesh	104	33	Pelvicol: 79% Gynemesh: 97%	Prospective/ retrospective cohort
Quiroz et al, 2008	Pelvicol, Autologous Fascia, Synthetic Mesh	259	13	Pelvicol: 89% Autologous Fascia: 93% Synthetic Mesh: 99%	Retrospective series

Definitions of cure and surgical technique vary for each study.
Adapted from Yurteri-Kaplan LA, Gutman RE. The use of biological materials in urogynecologic reconstruction: a systematic review. Plast Reconstr Surg 2012;130(5 Suppl 2):247S; with permission.

CARE trial (Colpopexy and Urinary Reduction Efforts) demonstrated that 71% to 76% of women had symptomatic relief of POP with abdominal SCP, and only 5% required re-treatment at 7 years follow-up.[5] The 2013 *Cochrane Review* included 56 randomized controlled trials (RCTs) and showed that SCP was associated with a lower rate of recurrent vault prolapse and lower reoperation rates than native tissue or transvaginal mesh (TVM) repairs.[6] Specifically, 3 trials showed no significant difference between the abdominal SCP and the sacrospinous ligament suspension with regard to subjective outcomes; however, recurrent vault prolapse was higher in the vaginal group.[7,8] Similarly, Rondini and colleagues[9] in 2015 demonstrated superiority of the SCP to vaginal uterosacral colpopexy with a higher objective success rate and lower reoperation rate. The operating time and postoperative complication rates were all higher for SCP than vaginal uterosacral colpopexy. Based on this evidence, abdominal SCP has been considered one of the gold standard surgical procedures for correction of apical prolapse, with high success rates and few complications.[6]

INTRODUCTION OF MINIMALLY INVASIVE SACRAL COLPOPEXY

With the proven success of the open SCP technique with polypropylene graft, it was inevitable that it would undergo the transformation to a more minimally invasive approach as surgical technology improved. In 1994, the first laparoscopic sacral colpopexy (LSCP) was described, touting the anticipated advantages of reduced morbidity, shorter hospital stay, and easier placement of posterior mesh arm along the posterior vaginal wall.[10] Then, in 2005, the FDA approved the daVinci robot for gynecologic surgery. Surgeons quickly adopted this approach because of the relatively fast learning curve associated with robotic compared with laparoscopic techniques. Today, with several trials demonstrating the utility of minimally invasive techniques, there is compelling evidence for the use of these approaches.

LEVEL 1 EVIDENCE FOR LAPAROSCOPIC SACROCOLPOPEXY

Freeman and colleagues[11] published the first RCT comparing open SCP to LSCP in 2013. In this multicenter equivalence trial, patients with grade 2 (Baden-Walker system) or greater posthysterectomy vaginal vault prolapse were randomized to either open or LSCP. Of the 27 open SCP and 26 LSCP patients, anatomic success (point "C" on the pelvic organ prolapse quantification [POP-Q]) was equivalent in both groups at 1 year. Both groups achieved subjective improvement on standardized quality-of-life scores at 1 year. LSCP had significantly less blood loss and shorter hospital stay, although there was no difference between groups in return to usual activities. No differences were seen in operative time or in the length of mesh extension along the posterior vaginal wall.[11] There were no mesh exposures seen at 1-year follow-up in either group, and no difference was seen in pelvic pain, constipation, or dyspareunia between the groups. This study provided level 1 evidence that LSCP provided equivalent outcomes to open SCP, with the additional advantage of reduced blood loss and shorter hospital stay.

COMPARISON OF SACRAL COLPOPEXY APPROACHES

The benefits of a minimally invasive approach to SCP are demonstrated in a multicenter retrospective cohort study comparing open abdominal SCP, LSCP, and robotic sacral colpopexy (RSCP).[12] Of 1124 patients, 535 (48%) had SCP via a minimally invasive technique: 273 (51%) LSCP and 262 (49%) RSCP. The open SCP group had longer hospitalizations and greater overall complication rates compared with the minimally invasive techniques. When comparing the laparoscopic and robotic approaches, anatomic outcomes as measured by POP-Q values were similar at an average of 8-months follow-up. RSCP had the benefit of fewer complications than LSCP (7% vs 18%; P<.02). However, RSCP took longer (316 vs 272 minutes; P<.001) and had a longer length of hospitalization than LSCP. The increased complication rate in the LSCP group compared was driven in part by the increased rate of conversion to laparotomy. The LSCP conversion rate was 2.4%, which is consistent with the literature for LSCP, but higher than the RSCP group. This finding may be partially explained by the definition of conversion set by the study: for conversion to be counted in the RSCP group, docking of the robot was required. Therefore, any planned RSCP cases that converted to open SCP due to adhesions before docking were counted as laparoscopic conversion, possibly skewing the data by attributing these complications to the LSCP group.[12]

LEVEL 1 EVIDENCE COMPARING ROBOTIC VERSUS LAPAROSCOPIC SACROCOLPOPEXY

Currently, there are 2 RCTs that compare RSCP to LSCP. The first trial randomized women with stage 2 to 4 posthysterectomy vault prolapse to either LSCP (38 patients) or RSCP (40 patients).[13] Both groups showed significant improvement 1 year postoperatively in vaginal support and functional outcomes. There was no difference in anatomic POP-Q measurements or subjective validated questionnaires between groups at 1-year follow-up. RSCP was shown to be significantly longer by approximately 1 hour, and patients had significantly more pain at rest and with activity in the early postoperative period (weeks 3–5), but this difference disappeared by the 6-week postoperative mark. A potential cause of increased discomfort could be attributed to the additional port and increased port size required for the robotic procedure (RSCP used two 12-mm ports and three 8-mm ports, while LSCP used two 5-mm and two 10/12-mm ports). One criticism of this study was that surgeons were more experienced in LSCP than RSCP, and the 2 primary surgeons were required to complete only 10 robotic cases before the trial. No difference was seen in intraoperative (cystostomy, enterotomy) or postoperative (infection, erosion, bowel obstruction) complication rates.[13]

The second RCT (Abdominal Colpopexy: Comparison of Endoscopic Surgical Strategies, ACCESS) looked primarily at cost of care as well as postoperative outcomes for LSCP versus RSCP.[14] Seventy-eight women with stage 2 or greater prolapse were randomized to LSCP (38 women) or RSCP (40 women). Surgical outcomes by POP-Q stage and symptom bother by validated questionnaire were equivalent at 6-months follow-up. The RSCP group had significantly longer operating room times (202.8 minutes compared with 178.4 minutes, P = .03) and higher pain scores 1 week after surgery, but this difference disappeared by the 2-week postoperative mark. There were no differences in the intraoperative complications. A criticism of the study is that surgeons had to have completed only 10 cases in the operative technique used, and that training-level surgeons participated.[14]

In summary, RCTs have shown no significant difference in objective or subjective outcomes between RSCP and LSCP. The minimally invasive approach, whether it be laparoscopic or robotic, is superior to the open SCP in regards to hospital stay and blood loss. Robotic surgery has allowed surgeons with less laparoscopic experience the opportunity to offer a minimally invasive approach to their patients, which has been shown to have benefits over the open approach. However, RSCP is associated with significantly higher cost and longer operating time than LSCP.

LAPAROSCOPIC MESH CONCLUSIONS

- Minimally invasive SCP offers the benefit of reduced blood loss and decreased length of stay compared with the open approach, without compromising anatomic or subjective outcomes.
- LSCP and RSCP have similar anatomic and subjective outcomes, but RSCP is associated with longer operative times and higher cost.

BACKGROUND ON TRANSVAGINAL MESH

TVM procedures were developed with the intent of improving anatomic cure rates of native tissue vaginal prolapse repairs. The first TVM product designed for POP was approved in 2004. In these procedures, synthetic polypropylene mesh is inserted transvaginally into the vesicovaginal and/or rectovaginal space, with the sacrospinous ligaments usually being used as an apical fixation point. These procedures are generally performed with kits that include delivery systems—often with specific trocars and fixation tips intended to hold the mesh in place once it is delivered. The idea for TVM procedures was predicated on evidence from the hernia literature, documenting improved cure rates when herniorrhaphy was performed with the addition of a synthetic graft.[15] TVM procedures were initially developed under the premise that combining the durability of mesh with the minimally invasive vaginal surgical approach would provide more longevity than native tissue repairs (NTRs) and reduced morbidity of open abdominal mesh procedures.

Initial case series of TVM reported high cure rates (>90%) and low risks of complications.[16] TVM kits, marketed heavily by manufacturers to urologists and gynecologists as a way to improve success rates of native tissue POP repairs, increased in popularity, and adoption of the technology was rapid.[17] According to 2010 data from the FDA, 25% of all POP surgeries in that year used TVM.[18]

Since the FDA approved the first TVM product for POP in 2004, much has changed. Unfortunately, the safety and efficacy of these kits were not adequately investigated before marketing, and after a rapid surge in TVM use, the FDA noted an increase in adverse events related to the TVM devices. Across the world, health care professionals and members of the public were reporting adverse events. The Medicines and Healthcare products Regulatory Agency (MHRA) in the United Kingdom noted most complications were related to mesh exposure (6%) and de novo dyspareunia (15%), similar results to those reported to the FDA (**Fig. 1**). In 2008, the FDA issued a public health notification to inform physicians and patients of these adverse events.[19] In the 3 years that followed, medical device reports related to TVM increased 5-fold, prompting the FDA to release a Safety Communication in 2011. The updated FDA warning stated that TVM was not routinely found to be more effective than NTR and may expose patients to greater risk.[20] These notifications brought confusion and concern regarding the use of TVM to health care providers and patients alike. In response, the American College of Obstetricians and Gynecologists and the American Urogynecologic Society released a Committee Opinion in December 2011 offering recommendations on the use of TVM: restricted use to high-risk patients, device-specific training to experienced reconstructive pelvic surgeons, adequate informed consent, and the need for continued surveillance of existing products as well as rigorous comparative trials between TVM and NTRs.[15]

In April 2014, the FDA proposed to reclassify TVM for POP from a class II (low to moderate-risk) to a class III (high-risk) device. (This reclassification does not include mesh for stress urinary incontinence or mesh for transabdominal POP repair such as sacral colpopexy.)[21] The FDA reclassification requires manufacturers of TVM to

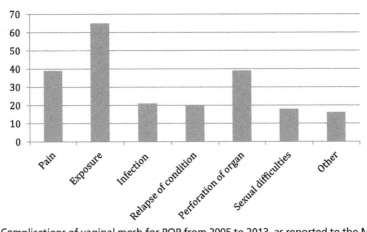

Fig. 1. Complications of vaginal mesh for POP from 2005 to 2013, as reported to the MHRA by health care professionals, members of the public, and manufacturers. Other complications include device-related complications (material or labeling issues), procedural complications (blood loss, rupture of iliac artery, or death), or postprocedural complications (fistula, thickening of vaginal skin). (*Adapted from* A summary of the evidence on the benefits and risks of vaginal mesh implants from the Medicines and Healthcare products Regulatory Agency (MHRA). Available at: https://www.gov.uk/government/uploads/system/uploads/attachment_data/file/402162/Summary_of_the_evidence_on_the_benefits_and_risks_of_vaginal_mesh_implants.pdf. Accessed October 28, 2014.)

obtain premarket approval for any new devices, requiring novel products to undergo rigorous testing compared with NTRs before their approval for use. At this point in time, after-market surveillance studies ("522 studies") are ongoing to better understand the long-term safety and effectiveness of TVM.

TRANSVAGINAL MESH FOR ANTERIOR WALL SUPPORT

Most currently available evidence for TVM use in POP repair surgeries evaluates its use in the anterior vaginal compartment—the most common site of prolapse. In the 2013 *Cochrane Review*, 10 trials compared native tissue with nonabsorbable synthetic TVM in the anterior wall. In one of the largest RCTs comparing native tissue anterior repair with TVM, Altman and colleagues[22] showed that TVM was superior to native tissue in anatomic and subjective cure at 1 year with composite success rates of 60.8% in the TVM compared with 34.5% in the native tissue group (95% confidence interval [CI] 15.6–37.0). Overall, the *Cochrane Review* showed that NTRs were associated with more recurrent anatomic prolapse than TVM repairs using polypropylene mesh (relative risk [RR] 3.15, 95% CI 2.50–3.96). In addition, women who underwent NTR of the anterior wall noted increased awareness of prolapse compared with polypropylene mesh (28% vs 18%, RR 1.57, 95% CI 1.18–2.07).

Despite the anatomic and subjective advantages of mesh in the anterior wall, reoperation rates for anterior wall prolapse were statistically similar between NTR (3%) and anterior polypropylene mesh repair (1.3%; RR 2.18, 95% CI 0.93–5.10).[6] Moreover, some data suggest that TVM for anterior wall prolapse is associated with higher overall reoperation rates than NTR. Using adjudicated health care claims of women who underwent traditional anterior colporrhaphy compared with TVM from 2005 to 2010, Jonsson Funk and colleagues[17] showed the 5-year cumulative risk of any repeat surgery to be significantly higher for TVM versus native tissue (15.2% vs 9.8%, *P*<.0001).

The 5-year risk of mesh revision/removal was 5.9%. Because the risk of surgery for recurrent prolapse was similar between groups (10.4% vs 9.3%, $P = .70$), their analysis indicated the higher reoperation rate seen in the TVM group was due to surgery for mesh complications, not for recurrent prolapse.

TRANSVAGINAL MESH FOR POSTERIOR PROLAPSE

Evidence does not support the use of any grafts at the time of posterior vaginal repair. Several trials have shown a similar rectocele recurrence rate with and without the use of several types of graft reinforcement. In a randomized trial comparing posterior repair with and without polyglactin, Sand and colleagues[23] showed no difference in rectocele recurrence. Similarly, porcine grafts have not shown a consistent advantage over native tissue posterior repair at 12 months.[24,25] Finally, in summarizing the 12 trials in the 2013 *Cochrane Review* comparing the use of nonabsorbable synthetic graft material in the posterior wall compared with traditional native tissue colporhhaphy, no advantage of mesh was found.

TRANSVAGINAL MESH FOR APICAL AND MULTICOMPARTMENT PROLAPSE

Few level 1 studies evaluate TVM use for apical and multicompartment prolapse. The 3-year outcomes of the Vaginal Mesh for Prolapse repair trial, a double-blind multicenter RCT, were published in 2013.[26] Women with stage 2 to 4 POP were treated with either a traditional NTR (anterior/posterior colporrhaphy plus vaginal colpopexy as indicated) or a vaginal mesh repair (anterior prolift or total prolift). All women with a uterus underwent vaginal hysterectomy. Using predetermined safety criteria, the trial was prematurely halted because of a mesh exposure rate of 15.6%. Before stopping the trial, 65 women were enrolled (33 mesh; 32 no mesh), with 51 women (78%) available at 3 years for quality-of-life assessment and 41 women (63%) that returned for pelvic examination at 2 to 3 years. The 3-year outcomes evaluated various definitions of cure (anatomic, symptomatic, and combined) and found no significant differences between the mesh and no mesh groups regardless of definition used. Composite cure was 65% for mesh and 57% for no mesh when the hymen was used as the threshold. Anatomic cure using no prolapse beyond hymen was 85% for mesh and 71% for no mesh. Symptomatic cure (92% mesh vs 81% no mesh) and satisfaction (88% mesh vs 81% no mesh) were high for both groups. No statistically significant differences were found between groups, possibly because the study was underpowered after it was halted early due to a high mesh exposure rate.[26]

In another randomized trial comparing laparoscopic SCP to TVM for apical prolapse, Maher and colleagues[27] assessed objective and subjective success 2 years postoperatively. They found objective success rates at all vaginal sites to be 41 of 53 (77%) for laparoscopic SCP versus 23 of 55 (43%) for vaginal mesh ($P<.001$). They also found a significantly higher reoperation rate associated with vaginal mesh surgery 12 of 55 (22%) compared with laparoscopic SCP of 3 of 53 (5%) ($P = .006$).

Similar to vaginal mesh use for anterior prolapse, evidence suggests a higher overall reoperation rate with TVM versus NTR when used for multicompartment prolapse—mostly due to mesh-related complications. In a review of complications and reoperation after apical repairs, vaginal mesh had a higher reoperation rate (8.5%) compared with native tissue vaginal repairs (3.2%).[28] This finding was similarly noted in the *Cochrane Review* for multicompartment treatment of prolapse. The reoperation rate after transvaginal polypropylene mesh repair (11%) was higher than after NTR (3.7%; RR 3.1, 95% CI 1.3–7.3).[6]

Currently, no studies show quality-of-life differences between mesh and NTRs, and quality of life may be the most important factor from a patient's perspective. Patient-centered outcomes research suggests that anatomic outcomes correlate poorly with patients' perception of success after prolapse surgery, and that the absence of a sensation of vaginal bulge, rather than anatomic success alone, impacts overall patient perception of improvement. The National Institutes of Health Pelvic Floor Disorders Network now recommends that subjective outcomes be included in the definition of success for surgery.[29]

In summary, TVM in the anterior wall has been shown to reduce anatomic failure rates compared with traditional anterior colporrhaphy as well as decrease the symptom of bulge. Current evidence does not support the use of TVM for apical, posterior, or multicompartment prolapse. In addition, no differences in quality of life have been shown between TVM and NTR repairs, even for anterior wall prolapse. Thus, the benefits of using TVM must be carefully weighed against the risks of its use. To determine the future value of these procedures, more extensive long-term composite outcome data for TVM products are needed.

TRANSVAGINAL MESH CONCLUSIONS

- TVM improves anatomic outcomes and sensation of bulge when used for repairs in the anterior compartment compared with NTR.
- Despite anatomic benefit in the anterior wall, TVM has not been shown to significantly improve quality of life.
- Because of the known complications associated with TVM use (dyspareunia, mesh exposure or erosion), TVM prolapse repairs may best be used on-protocol.
- There is currently no evidence for use of TVM in apical, posterior, or multicompartment POP.

SUMMARY

Synthetic mesh may be placed abdominally or transvaginally during prolapse repair surgery. The SCP procedure with abdominally placed synthetic mesh is generally considered the gold standard surgical procedure for apical POP. The minimally invasive SCP is an alternative approach to this procedure, providing comparable anatomic and subjective outcomes with the benefit of reduced blood loss and decreased hospital length of stay. Surgeons have quickly adopted robotics for SCP due to its perceived advantages of improved ergonomics, rapid learning curve, and advanced instrument articulation; however, at this time, no RCT has identified a difference with regard to anatomic or subjective outcomes for RSCP compared with LSCP. Although the minimally invasive approach to SCP has proven benefits, more research is needed to further define the specific role of robotics in a health care environment focused on outcomes and efficiency.

TVM procedures were initially designed to augment native tissue and reduce the morbidity of open abdominal mesh procedures. In appropriately selected patients, synthetic TVM can improve anatomic cure rates in the anterior compartment; however, most studies fail to show a significant improvement in quality of life when comparing TVM with native tissue vaginal repairs in any compartment. Because of the potential complications associated with TVM, appropriate patient selection and counseling are imperative, and many consider the use of TVM best reserved for on-protocol use at this time. Ultimately, the results of the prospective FDA 522 trials comparing TVM to NTRs over a long-term follow-up will help to determine the future use of TVM.

REFERENCES

1. Dieter AA, Wilkins MF, Wu JM. Epidemiological trends and future care needs for pelvic floor disorders. Curr Opin Obstet Gynecol 2015;27(5):380–4.
2. Samuelsson EC, Victor A, Tibblin G, et al. Signs of genital prolapse in a Swedish population of women 20 to 59 years of age and possible related factors. Am J Obstet Gynecol 1999;180(2 Pt 1):299–305.
3. Nygaard IE, McCreery R, Brubaker L, et al. Abdominal sacrocolpopexy: a comprehensive review. Obstet Gynecol 2004;104(4):805–23.
4. Yurteri-Kaplan LA, Gutman RE. The use of biological materials in urogynecologic reconstruction: a systematic review. Plast Reconstr Surg 2012;130(5 Suppl 2): 242S–53S.
5. Nygaard I, Brubaker L, Zyczynski HM, et al. Long-term outcomes following abdominal sacrocolpopexy for pelvic organ prolapse. JAMA 2013;309(19):2016–24.
6. Maher C, Feiner B, Baessler K, et al. Surgical management of pelvic organ prolapse in women [review]. Cochrane Database Syst Rev 2013;(4):CD004014.
7. Benson JT, Lucente V, McClellan E. Vaginal versus abdominal reconstructive surgery for the treatment of pelvic support defects: a prospective randomized study with long-term outcome evaluation. Am J Obstet Gynecol 1996;175(6):1418–21.
8. Maher CF, Qatawneh AM, Dwyer PL, et al. Abdominal sacral colpopexy or vaginal sacrospinous colpopexy for vaginal vault prolapse: a prospective randomized study. Am J Obstet Gynecol 2004;190(1):20–6.
9. Rondini C, Braun H, Alvarez J, et al. High uterosacral vault suspension vs. Sacrocolpopexy for treating apical defects: a randomized controlled trial with twelve months follow-up. Int Urogynecol J 2015;26(8):1131–8.
10. Nezhat CH, Nezhat F, Nezhat C. Laparoscopic sacral colpopexy for vaginal vault prolapse. Obstet Gynecol 1994;84(5):885–8.
11. Freeman RM, Pantazis K, Thomson A, et al. A randomised controlled trial of abdominal versus laparoscopic sacrocolpopexy for the treatment of posthysterectomy vaginal vault prolapse: LAS study. Int Urogynecol J Pelvic Floor Dysfunct 2013;24(3):377–84.
12. Nosti PA, Umoh Andy U, Kane S, et al. Outcomes of abdominal and minimally invasive sacrocolpopexy: a retrospective cohort study. Female Pelvic Med Reconstr Surg 2014;20(1):33–7.
13. Paraiso MFR, Jelovsek JE, Frick A, et al. Laparoscopic compared with robotic sacrocolpopexy for vaginal prolapse. Obstet Gynecol 2011;118(5):1005–13.
14. Anger JT, Mueller ER, Tarnay C, et al. Robotic compared with laparoscopic sacrocolpopexy: a randomized controlled trial. Obstet Gynecol 2014;123(1):5–12.
15. American College of Obstetricians and Gynecologists. Committee Opinion no. 513: vaginal placement of synthetic mesh for pelvic organ prolapse. Obstet Gynecol 2011;118(6):1459–64.
16. De Tayrac R, Gervaise A, Chauveaud A, et al. Tension-free polypropylene mesh for vaginal repair of anterior vaginal wall prolapse. J Reprod Med 2005;50(2):75–80.
17. Jonsson Funk M, Edenfield AL, Pate V, et al. Trends in use of surgical mesh for pelvic organ prolapse. Am J Obstet Gynecol 2013;208(1):79.e1–7.
18. Urogynecologic surgical mesh: update on the safety and effectiveness of transvaginal placement for pelvic organ prolapse. Available at: http://www.fda.gov/downloads/medicaldevices/safety/alertsandnotices/UCM262760.pdf. Accessed May 6, 2014; Accessed September 10, 2015.
19. Health C for D and R. Public Health Notifications (Medical Devices) - FDA Public Health Notification: Serious Complications Associated with Transvaginal Placement

of Surgical Mesh in Repair of Pelvic Organ Prolapse and Stress Urinary Incontinence. Available at: http://www.fda.gov/MedicalDevices/Safety/AlertsandNotices/PublicHealthNotifications/ucm061976.htm. Accessed September 10, 2015.

20. Health C for D and R. Safety Communications - UPDATE on Serious Complications Associated with Transvaginal Placement of Surgical Mesh for Pelvic Organ Prolapse: FDA Safety Communication. Available at: http://www.fda.gov/MedicalDevices/Safety/AlertsandNotices/ucm262435.htm. Accessed September 10, 2015.

21. Reclassification of Surgical Mesh for Transvaginal Pelvic Organ Prolapse Repair and Surgical Instrumentation for Urogynecologic Surgical Mesh Procedures; Designation of Special Controls for Urogynecologic Surgical Mesh Instrumentation. Available at: https://www.federalregister.gov/articles/2014/05/01/2014-09907/reclassification-of-surgical-mesh-for-transvaginal-pelvic-organ-prolapse-repair-and-surgical. Accessed September 10, 2015.

22. Altman D, Väyrynen T, Engh ME, et al. Anterior colporrhaphy versus transvaginal mesh for pelvic-organ prolapse. Int Braz J Urol 2011;37(5):675.

23. Sand PK, Koduri S, Lobel RW, et al. Prospective randomized trial of polyglactin 910 mesh to prevent recurrence of cystoceles and rectoceles. Am J Obstet Gynecol 2001;184:1357–64.

24. Paraiso MFR, Barber MD, Muir TW, et al. Rectocele repair: a randomized trial of three surgical techniques including graft augmentation. Am J Obstet Gynecol 2006;195(6):1762–71.

25. Sung VW, Rardin CR, Raker CA, et al. Porcine subintestinal submucosal graft augmentation for rectocele repair. Obstet Gynecol 2012;119(1):125–33.

26. Gutman RE, Nosti Pa, Sokol AI, et al. Three-year outcomes of vaginal mesh for prolapse: a randomized controlled trial. Obstet Gynecol 2013;122(4):770–7.

27. Maher CF, Feiner B, DeCuyper EM, et al. Laparoscopic sacral colpopexy versus total vaginal mesh for vaginal vault prolapse: a randomized trial. Am J Obstet Gynecol 2011;204(4):360.e1–7.

28. Diwadkar GB, Barber MD, Feiner B, et al. Complication and reoperation rates after apical vaginal prolapse surgical repair: a systematic review. Obstet Gynecol 2009;113(2 Pt 1):367–73.

29. Barber MD, Brubaker L, Nygaard I, et al. Defining success after surgery for pelvic organ prolapse. Obstet Gynecol 2009;114(3):600–9.

Evidence-Based Update on Treatments of Fecal Incontinence in Women

Isuzu Meyer, MD*, Holly E. Richter, PhD, MD

KEYWORDS

- Accidental bowel leakage • Anal incontinence • Anal sphincter
- Defecatory disorders • Fecal incontinence • Treatment • Surgical treatment

KEY POINTS

- Fecal incontinence (FI), defined as the complaint of involuntary loss of liquid and/or solid stool, is caused by disruption of the multicomponent continence mechanism.
- FI is a physically and psychosocially debilitating condition. Many women are reluctant to report their symptoms and seek care.
- Management options for FI consist of conservative and/or surgical approaches, and more-invasive therapies should be reserved for patients with a refractory condition.
- Traditionally, options were limited once patients had failed conservative therapies. Surgical management of FI was considered invasive and provided only short-term success with high complication rates.
- Recent research has demonstrated not only the long-term safety and efficacy data on existing modalities but also the development of less-invasive options and investigational devices.

INTRODUCTION

FI, defined as the complaint of involuntary loss of liquid and/or solid stool, is a highly prevalent condition. In community-dwelling women, the reported prevalence of FI varies widely from 2.2% to 24% and rises with advancing age.[1–8] Epidemiologic studies suggest that up to 70% of patients with FI have not reported their symptoms to health care professionals.[9,10] Thus, the prevalence of FI is often underestimated. The negative

Financial Disclosure: None (I. Meyer); Grant Support: Partially supported by the National Institutes of Diabetes and Digestive and Kidney Diseases, 2K24-DK068389; Consultant: Kimberly Clark and Pelvalon; Royalties: UpToDate (H.E. Richter).
Conflict of Interest: None.
Division of Urogynecology and Pelvic Reconstructive Surgery, Department of Obstetrics and Gynecology, University of Alabama at Birmingham, 1700 6th Avenue South, Suite 10382, Birmingham, AL 35233, USA
* Corresponding author.
E-mail address: imeyer@uabmc.edu

consequences of FI include not only the physical debilitation but also the social isolation, embarrassment, loss of employment, and effect on intimate relationships and self-esteem. To reduce the burden of FI, eliminate stigma, and promote care-seeking, it is important to raise public awareness of the condition and various treatment options available to those who suffer in silence. Another obstacle to help-seeking is that many providers fail to screen for FI because of the complexity in evaluation as well as a lack of clinical experience and knowledge on the current management approaches.

The etiology of FI is multifactorial and caused by the disruption of the continence mechanism dependent on anal sphincter function, intact rectal sensation, adequate rectal capacity, compliance, colonic transit time, stool consistency, and cognitive and neurologic factors. It was reported that 80% of patients with FI had more than 1 continence factor compromised.[11] This article reviews the evidence-based approach in the management of FI.

MANAGEMENT

The goal of treatment should focus on restoring continence and improving quality of life (QOL). Health care providers should routinely ask patients about the presence of FI directly, rather than relying on voluntary reporting, and identify conditions and risk factors that may predispose to FI. To provide proper treatment, clinicians should determine symptom severity and characterize stool type, frequency, amount of leakage, and the presence of urgency. It is helpful to obtain bowel diaries because they are shown superior to self-reports for characterizing bowel habits and can better predict colonic transit.[12,13] Recognizing the type of FI based on the awareness of the desire to defecate before leakage can provide clues to underlying pathology: (1) urgency incontinence, or inability to postpone defecation on urgency, can be related to external anal sphincter (EAS) dysfunction; (2) passive incontinence, or the loss of stool without the urge to defecate, is often attributed to internal anal sphincter (IAS) dysfunction and peripheral neuropathy; and (3) fecal seepage is related to incomplete evacuation and impaired rectal sensation.

Management of FI consists of conservative and surgical approaches. Conservative treatment includes lifestyle changes, medications, pelvic floor muscle exercises, physical therapy with or without biofeedback. Unfortunately, no single option has been shown to provide consistent, long-term effectiveness with low complication rates, making FI extremely difficult to manage. However, symptoms may be alleviated by simple measures.

Dietary Considerations

Avoid offending foods

The frequency and consistency of stool can greatly affect symptom severity. Patients should be educated on factors contributing to bowel disturbances and loose stool consistency, including foods containing incompletely digested sugars (fructose and lactose), sweeteners (sorbitol, xylitol, and mannitol), carbonated beverages, caffeine, alcohol, cured or smoked meat (sausage, ham, and turkey), spicy foods, and fatty/greasy foods. Bowel and food diaries can help identify an individual's offending food items that cause loose stools and incontinence. In cases of diarrhea, patients should be evaluated and treated for any underlying cause. Fecal impaction should be treated and prevent further constipation to avoid overflow incontinence.

Fiber supplementation

Fiber supplementation along with dietary modification is one of the first-line treatment options for FI, which is helpful particularly in women with low-volume, loose-stool–associated FI. The mechanisms of dietary fiber depend on stool composition and consistency, which vary among the types of fiber ingested. Fiber, when fermented but not completely degraded by colonic bacteria, has been shown to increase stool bulk. In addition, fiber with high water-holding capacity allows a gel formation that normalizes stool consistency (softens hard stool and firms loose/liquid stool). Insoluble fiber increases fecal water content and bulking, however, accelerates colonic transit rate, thus having a laxative effect. Increasing rectal distension can improve sensory awareness of the need to defecate, which may reduce FI episodes and promote complete evacuation of stool, leaving less in the rectum to leak.[11,14,15] Compared with constipation, data on the effects of fiber supplementation on FI are limited, and most studies are not adequately powered.

Commonly used fiber supplements include methylcellulose (Citrucel [GlaxoSmithKline, Middlesex, United Kingdom]: high solubility and nonfermentable), psyllium (Metamucil [Procter & Gamble, Cincinnati, OH]: moderate solubility and fermentable), and calcium polycarbophil (Fibercon [Pfizer, New York, NY]: an insoluble hydrophilic fiber).[16,17] A recent placebo-controlled study compared the effect of dietary fiber supplements (carboxymethylcelulose, gum arabic, and psyllium) based on the different levels of fermentability/solubility versus placebo in subjects with loose/liquid stool–associated FI. After the 32-day treatment period, psyllium significantly decreased FI episodes compared with the placebo or other fiber groups. The studies further analyzed the characteristics of feces. Of the 4 groups, psyllium had the highest total fiber content, suggesting that the fermented psyllium products are not completely degraded. In addition, a gel formation was found only in the feces of the psyllium group, maintaining stool consistency.[14]

Recommended total dietary fiber intake is 25 to 35 grams per day for adults. Fiber should be added to the diet slowly to avoid bloating. Because of the bulking nature, fiber could exacerbate symptoms in women with decreased compliance (radiation, prior surgery, or proctitis).

Medications

Antidiarrheal medications have been shown to improve symptoms of diarrhea-associated FI. Loperamide (Imodium) is a synthetic opioid that inhibits intestinal peristalsis increasing oral-cecal transit time. Loperamide can increase resting anal sphincter tone and improve rectal perception and rectal compliance.[18] Compared with placebo, loperamide was more effective for reducing urgency FI, with more people achieving full continence, improved symptoms, and fewer FI episodes.[19] Loperamide has fewer central nervous system side effects compared with diphenoxylate/atropine (Lomotil).[20] A recent randomized double-blind placebo-controlled crossover trial examined the effectiveness of loperamide versus psyllium fiber for reducing FI episodes. In this study, participants received either daily loperamide (plus placebo psyllium powder) or psyllium powder (plus loperamide placebo) for 4 weeks (first treatment), followed by a 2-week washout period, and then crossed over to the other treatment for additional 4 weeks (second treatment). A significant reduction in FI episodes per week was found in both groups compared with baseline (loperamide 7.9–7.1, $P<0.001$; psyllium 7.3–4.8, $P = 0.008$). The number of FI episodes was similar, however, between the loperamide first and psyllium first groups, both at the end of first and second treatments. In addition, both interventions improved symptom severity and QOL. The overall rate of adverse events was similar between the groups; however, constipation was seen more in the loperamide group (29% loperamide vs 10% psyllium).[21] Currently, a randomized controlled trial (RCT) using loperamide (Controlling Anal incontinence by Performing Anal Exercises with Biofeedback or Loperamide [CAPABLe]) is being undertaken by the Pelvic Floor Disorders Network (National Institutes of Health [NIH], NCT02008565). This trial, using a factorial design, compares the use of loperamide to oral placebo and the use of anal sphincter exercise training with biofeedback to usual care (basic education with pamphlet) in the treatment of women suffering from FI.[22]

Cholestyramine (2–6 g daily) can be helpful as an adjunct therapy, especially in patients with bile salt malabsorption.[16,23,24] Anticholinergic medications, such as hyoscyamine, 0.125 mg to 0.25 mg, if taken 30 to 60 minutes before meals, are thought helpful in postprandial leakage. Hyoscyamine induces relaxation of intestinal smooth muscles and decreases gastric acid secretions. The use of hyoscyamine, however, outside of clinical experience is supported by little evidence with lack of placebo-controlled studies.[25] Given dose-dependent adverse events related to anticholinergics (dry mouth, dizziness and blurred vision, fatigue, and constipation), this medication should be avoided in the elderly.

Amitriptyline has been shown to prolong colon transit time by decreasing rectal contractions in patients with idiopathic FI.[16,17] Clonidine, an α_2-adrenergic agonist, 0.1 mg twice daily, has been also used for treatment of FI. A recent RCT on urgency-predominant FI reported, however, that clonidine did not affect bowel symptoms, fecal continence, or anorectal functions compared with placebo. Among patients with diarrhea, clonidine increased stool consistency and decreased diarrheal episodes but not FI frequency.[26] Topical phenylephrine can increase smooth muscle tone and has been evaluated on patients with FI associated with decreased IAS tone. The results were statistically significant; however, only weak improvements in FI symptoms were shown. The current evidence is inconclusive to recommend this therapy.[16,19,27] Localized dermatitis or burning sensation, although short-lasting, have been observed.[19] The currently available supplements/medications and their level of evidence on treatment of FI are listed in **Table 1**.

Table 1
Current evidence on medical treatment of fecal incontinence

Medication	Suggested Dose	Level of Evidence[b]	Recommendation Grade[c]
Fiber supplementation	2–6 g[a]	II	B
Loperamide	2–4 mg per dose up to 16 mg/d	II	B
Diphynoxylate (with atropine)	2.5–5 mg (0.025 mg) per dose up to 20 mg/d	II	B
Cholestyramine	2–6 g/d	III	C
Hyoscyamine	0.125–0.25 mg before meal	III	C
Amitryptyline	20 mg nightly	II	B
Clonidine	0.1 mg twice daily	II	C
Phenylephrine topical	2.5-cm application of 10%–30% gel shown to have a therapeutic effect at 1 h	II	C

[a] Suggested total daily intake for adults is 25 to 35 grams.
[b] I: $\geq$1 properly RCT available; II: evidence based on well-designed cohort or retrospective case-controlled studies; and III: the evidence based on expert opinion or descriptive studies, case reports.
[c] A: strongly recommended; B: recommended; and C: evidence is not sufficient to recommend for or against the therapy.

Pelvic Floor Muscle Exercises and Biofeedback

Pelvic muscle exercises and biofeedback alleviate FI symptoms by improving contraction of the pelvic floor muscles, sensory-motor coordination required for continence, and enhancing the ability to perceive rectal distension.[28] Pelvic floor muscle training is recommended to nearly all patients with FI; however, no consensus exists on exercise regimen (ie, number, intensity, and duration of squeezing). The data on pre- and post-treatment comparisons of pelvic floor muscle exercises for FI are less established compared with urinary incontinence.

Biofeedback is performed using an anorectal manometry or surface electromyography. Biofeedback therapy focuses on 3 main targets. (1) The first is rectal sensitivity training: gradually distending a rectal balloon with air or water to determine the sensation of rectal filling. In patients with higher threshold, the training should focus on feeling the distention at lower volume to give a signal to get to the toilet sooner or squeeze muscles to prevent leakage, whereas if the patient has a low threshold (low-capacity, hypersensitive rectum), the goal is to focus on tolerating larger volumes. (2) The second is strength training: visual or auditory signals are used as a guidance to demonstrate the proper muscle isolation and improve squeeze pressures. (3) The third is coordination training: focusing on coordinating rectal distention and anal sphincter contraction. The goal is to achieve a maximum sphincter squeeze in less than 1 second after a rectal balloon is inflated to prevent leakage. Currently, there is no standardization of biofeedback treatment, likely contributing to the wide range in reported success rates of exercises with or without biofeedback, from 38% to as high as 100%.[11,29,30] Some studies have shown no major benefit for biofeedback, whereas more recent RCTs have favored the addition of biofeedback to pelvic floor muscle training.[29,31–33] Factors associated with worse outcomes for biofeedback include severe FI; pudendal neuropathy; underlying neurologic conditions; overflow incontinence associated with behavioral/psychiatric disorders; decreased rectal capacity from resection, inflammation, or fibrosis; and major structural damage to continence mechanisms. Biofeedback seems more beneficial in patients with urgency FI and useful in postsphincteroplasty or anal repair.[11,29] The American College of Gastroenterology and American Gastroenterological Association recognize biofeedback as a safe and effective approach and recommend its use especially in patients with weak sphincters and/or impaired rectal sensation.[11,30] A recent NIH consensus statement concluded that biofeedback is effective in preventing and reversing pregnancy-related FI for the first year after delivery; however, long-term data for the benefit of biofeedback on prevention are still lacking.[34] Further research should focus on standardizing optimal therapy regimens and guidelines.

Surgical Management

Significant innovative changes in the surgical treatment of FI have recently emerged. Existing studies vary, however, in the primary outcome measured (QOL, dichotomous continent/incontinent, and number of leakage episodes), making the interpretation and comparison of the results more challenging. In general, surgery should be offered to patients who have failed a credible attempt of conservative therapies.

Traditional approaches

Sphincteroplasty The most common cause of FI is EAS disruption, often noted in the anterior segment.[35] Delayed repair of anal sphincter disruption remote from delivery is reviewed. For most women, sphincter injuries are caused by obstetric trauma. The causes of chronic sphincter disruptions can be either unrecognized injuries at the time of childbirth, from a perineal repair breakdown, or persistent injuries after the primary repair. Among women who had a sphincter laceration repaired at the time of delivery, 35% continued to have IAS gaps; of those women, the majority had concomitant EAS disruptions noted on endoanal ultrasound at 6 to 12 months postpartum.[36]

The traditional sphincteroplasty is performed via a curvilinear incision made in the perineum on the outer edge of the EAS in the plane between the rectum and vagina.[37,38] To avoid pudendal nerve injury posteriorly, care should be taken not to extend the dissection laterally beyond 180° circumference of the anus. The sphincter muscles are typically divided through scar anteriorly if present, then plicated in an overlapping fashion to narrow the canal. When disrupted, both internal and external sphincters are mobilized together to create the overlapping repair. Separate dissection of the internal and external sphincters does not seem to provide better functions postoperatively.[39,40] Levator muscle plication has been shown to improve functional outcomes; however, it may cause significant dyspareunia in women.[41–43]

Sphincter plication has been shown effective at least in the short term.[35,44] Initially, 70% to 80% of patients reported symptom improvement. Long-term success rates deteriorate over time, however, ranging from 20% to 67% by 5 years, and even lower (0%–40%) at 10 years.[35,45–47] Bravo Gutierrez and colleagues[48] demonstrated a 6% complete continence rate at 10 years in their long-term study with 130 patients. In the same population, the incontinence rate increased from 36% at 3 years to 57% at 10 years. The existing data on the long-term efficacy of sphincteroplasty, as noted in a recent systematic review, are shown in **Fig. 1**. The most common complication is wound infection, ranging from 2% to 35%. Deep infection resulted in poor long-term outcomes.[44,45,49] Other factors of long-term failure include advanced age at the time of repair, duration of FI symptoms, and pudendal neuropathy, although controversial.[44,49] Preoperative anorectal manometry and endoanal ultrasonography have a limited role in predicting surgical success.[11] Nonetheless, diagnosis of a sphincter defect on imaging studies, most commonly with endoanal ultrasound, is warranted prior to sphincteroplasty.[49]

Special population: obstetric anal sphincter injuries

Pregnancy and childbirth are unique risk factors for FI in women. Two mechanisms of sphincter injury are either traction pudendal neuropathy or anatomic disruption of the

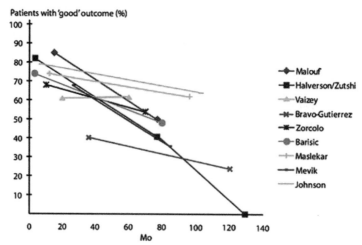

Fig. 1. Long-term efficacy outcomes of sphincteroplasty. (*From* Glasgow SC, Lowry AC. Long-term outcomes of anal sphincter repair for fecal incontinence: a systematic review. Dis Colon Rectum 2012;55:487. Wolters Kluwer Health, Inc; with permission.)

anal sphincter complex. Obstetric anal sphincter injuries (OASIS) from laceration or episiotomy at the time of vaginal delivery are strongly associated with FI, both immediate and delayed. In primiparous women, approximately 35% had sphincter defects noted on endoanal ultrasound at 6 to 8 weeks after vaginal delivery.[50] Many women with OASIS, however, do not develop FI symptoms until 2 to 3 decades after the initial insult.[51] The evidence for the optimal management in preventing OASIS is limited. The role of primary cesarean delivery to prevent OASIS is controversial. Both long-term follow-up data (5–12 years) and large population meta-analyses (12,000–31,500 women) showed no difference between spontaneous vaginal delivery versus cesarean section in preventing FI, whereas operative vaginal delivery and medial episiotomy are well-documented risk factors for OASIS.[52–56] The issue is often complicated in women with prior OASIS to determine the mode of delivery in the subsequence delivery. The risk of repeat OASIS with vaginal delivery has been reported as 4% to 8%.[57,58] Currently, the American College of Obstetricians and Gynecologists does not suggest primary elective cesarean delivery for prevention of FI (grade 2C) because planned cesarean delivery conferred no protection against FI.[59] In women with a history of FI or OASIS, data on the optimal mode of delivery for subsequent pregnancies are limited. Many experts advise that a woman with persistent FI and a poorly functioning anal sphincter be offered a planned cesarean for subsequent deliveries only after discussing the risks and benefits of both options and understanding the lack of data on this matter.[60,61]

In regard to third-degree and fourth-degree obstetric laceration repairs at the time of delivery, the existing data comparing overlapping versus end-to-end repair are conflicting. For the immediate repair with no scar present, most studies showed that the 2 approaches do not differ in surgical outcomes.[46,47] More recently, the randomized trial by Farrell and colleagues[62] reported that end-to-end repairs of complete third-degree and fourth-degree obstetric lacerations are associated with significantly lower rates of anal incontinence at 12 months. No differences, however, were observed over 3 years.

Neosphincter construction
In patients with severe refractory FI due to structural damage, such as complete perineal disruption from massive trauma or infection, neosphincter construction has been attempted either from autologous gracilis muscle or an artificial bowel sphincter.

Graciloplasty A slinglike structure is constructed using a patient's own gracilis muscle with 1 end attached to the pubis, encircling the anus, and the other end reattached to the opposite ischial tuberosity. A pulse generator (available in Europe but not in the United States) can be implanted to transform a fast-twitch skeletal muscle (fatigue-prone) into a slow-twitch muscle (fatigue-resistant) providing a sustained sphincter-like response.[11,63] Clinical success rates of 38% to 90% have been reported. However, gracilis muscle transfer has drawbacks, such as deterioration in effectiveness over time, a long learning curve for surgeons, and high morbidity. The complications include infection (28%), problems related to the device (15%), and leg pain (13%).[64] The revision rate due to major complications was up to 50%.[11] The muscle does not function as a dynamic sphincter; thus, evacuating feces can be challenging. Up to 90% of patients reported constipation or difficulty evacuation.[65] An overall mortality of 2% (0%–13%) was reported.[64]

Artificial bowel sphincter The currently available artificial bowel sphincter (ABS) consists of an inflatable cuff implanted around the anal canal with a pressure-regulating balloon placed in the prevesical space and a pump in the labia connecting the cuff and balloon. Patients can inflate the cuff to prevent stool passage and deflate to allow defecation. Existing data on the success rates and safety vary considerably. The largest study with 52 patients with a mean follow-up of 64 months reported the median Wexner Fecal Incontinence Score decreased significantly after ABS implantation even though full continence was rarely achieved.[66] Defecatory difficulties or constipation are not uncommon, however, with reported rates ranging from 6% to 83%.[66,67] The overall revision rate was 13% to 50%; however, cumulative risk of revision increases over time from 7% at 1 year, 40% to 60% at 5 years, and eventually reaching a plateau of approximately 90% after 5 to 10 years.[66–68] In addition, the explantation rates also increase overtime, 20% at 1 to 3 years to 40% at greater than or equal to 5 years.[66] The most common reason for surgical revision was device malfunction, such as micro-perforation and leak from the cuff because repeated inflation and deflation often causes cuff fatigue. Device erosion and infection are the most common reasons for device explantation.[68] Given the high morbidity, revision, and explantation rates, the use of ABS is currently limited, mostly for the treatment of end-stage severe FI.

Neuromodulation

Sacral neurostimulation

Sacral neurostimulation (SNS) was first introduced in Europe in 1995 as a minimally invasive treatment of FI.[69] The InterStim (Medtronic, Minneapolis, Minnesota) was approved by the US Food and Drug Administration (FDA) for treatment of chronic refractory FI in April 2011. The electrode is inserted typically in the S3 foramen to provide low-amplitude electrical current via a battery-operated stimulator. Proposed mechanisms of action include that SNS acts through a somato-visceral reflex pathway to reduce colonic activity and change rectal sensitivity, a direct effect on the anal sphincter complex to increase sphincter tone and reduce spontaneous sphincter relaxation, or afferent nerve modulation to improve compliance.[70–73] Improvements in FI symptoms, however, without changing sphincter pressures have also been reported.[70,74,75] Although data are limited, SNS has been shown effective in patients even with disrupted anal sphincters, including previously failed sphincteroplasty. The extent of sphincter gap differs in existing data; up to 180° sphincter separation has been studied. Treatment outcomes seem independent of size, although the results are less predictable, and effect sizes are smaller in these studies.[69,76–78] A few studies evaluated the efficacy of SNS in patients with neurogenic bowel (FI due to nerve injury or neurologic conditions), and SNS seems effective even in patients with neurologic disorders. Long-term data, however, are lacking.[79,80]

SNS is a 2-step procedure: (1) the testing phase with a temporary external neurostimulator and (2) placement of a battery-operated implantable pulse generator. For the testing phase, the staged trial technique with a permanent lead placement is preferred to the percutaneous nerve evaluation (PNE) using a temporary monopolar lead. Some providers use the PNE approach because this can be done in the office with local anesthesia; however, it is more prone to incorrect lead placement and lead migration (especially in obese or active patients), resulting in high false-negative rates. In addition, the PNE testing phase is typically 4 to 7 days, whereas the use of a permanent lead in a staged procedure allows a longer testing period, usually 2 to 4 weeks for the evaluation of FI treatment. Studies have shown high progression rates to implantable pulse generator implantation with the staged procedure using a permanent lead.[81] Batteries must be replaced approximately 7 years after implantation.

In a pivotal US multicenter trial, including 133 patients undergoing InterStim procedure, in 2010, 90% had a successful test stimulation and proceeded to the permanent implantation. At 12 months, 83% of the patients achieved therapeutic success, and

41% had complete continence. Incontinence episodes decreased from 9.4 episodes per week at baseline to 1.9 at 12 months and to 2.9 at 24 months.[82] This trial was extended, and the long-term results of SNS were published in 2013. Of the initial subjects, 63% (n = 76/120) were available for greater than or equal to 5-year follow-up. FI episodes per week were 1.7 at 5 years, with 89% of the subjects having greater than or equal to 50% symptomatic improvement, with 36% having complete continence.[83] Most studies define success as a greater than or equal to 50% reduction in FI episodes per week. When reviewing short-term (<12 months), medium-term (12–36 months), and long-term (>36 months) success for SNS, the median rates (range) were 63% (33–66), 58% (52–81), and 54% (50–58) per intention-to-treat (ITT) analysis compared with the median per-protocol rates of 79% (69–83), 80% (65–88), and 84% (75–100), respectively. Sustained clinical benefit of up to 14 years has been demonstrated in greater than 80% of subjects.[84] Existing data on the efficacy of medium-term to long-term follow-up studies are listed in **Table 2**.

Most adverse events (67%) occurred within the first year of implantation, and the majority required none to minimal interventions, such as medications. Common device-related adverse events are implant site pain (28%), paresthesia (15%), and changes in the sensation of stimulation (12%).[85] A recent meta-analysis, however, reported a lower rate of implant site pain of 6%.[86] Pain is usually managed conservatively by reprogramming of the device, medication, or no treatment. In some cases, revision or explantation of the neurostimulator and/or the lead may be required.[85–88] With advancements in the lead design and techniques, explantation of the device is rarely necessary (on average 3%–4%).[86,89] The infection rate is typically 3%; however, up to 11% has been reported.[82,85,90] Because of the minimally invasive surgical technique, high success rates, and minimal morbidity with no mortality, the current data suggest that SNS is an effective approach for treatment of FI.[69,90–92] Future studies should also explore the efficacy of SNS on patients not limited to intact sphincters as well as patients with neurogenic disorders for broader applicability.[93]

One of the concerns with the InterStim system is the use of MRI. The InterStim system has been shown MRI conditional based on nonclinical testing. Not all InterStim devices are MRI safe: all models of 3058 neurostimulators (InterStimII) are MRI eligible, whereas some of the 3023 (InterStim) models are not. The non-MRI–eligible series numbers are found in the MRI Guidelines for InterStim Therapy neurostimulation systems (Medtronic). Patients with MRI-eligible neurostimulators can undergo a certain head MRI scan (1.5-T horizontal closed bore with radiofrequency [RF] transmit head coil only). The neurostimulator needs to be turned off prior to examination. Patients during test stimulation or having any neurostimulation system components not fully implanted should not undergo MRI. It is important to discuss the risks of undergoing MRI with patients prior to implantation.

The safety and efficacy of SNS in pregnancy, the unborn fetus, and delivery have not been established. Existing data on SNS in pregnancy are derived from a retrospective study or case series with a small number of women with urinary complaints.[94,95] Due to lack of evidence, those who are considering or during pregnancy should turn off their neurostimulator.

Percutaneous tibial nerve stimulation

Percutaneous tibial nerve stimulation (PTNS) for FI has been approved in Europe but is under investigation in the United States. The PTNS treatment uses a 34-gauge needle as an electrode to stimulate the posterior tibial nerve near the medial malleolus to achieve effects via L4-S3 nerve roots. PTNS is a minimally invasive outpatient therapy with almost no associated morbidity. The reported estimated cost is less than one-

Table 2
Sacral neuromodulation efficacy in medium-term to long-term follow-up studies

Author, Year	Median Follow-up	Number of Subjects	Fecal Incontinence Episodes per Week		Greater Than or Equal to 50% Reduction in Fecal Incontinence Episodes (%)		Complete Continence (%)	
			Baseline	Post-therapy	Per Protocol	Intention to Treat	Per Protocol	Intention to Treat
Matzel et al,[88] 2004	24	30	16	2	88	81	35	32
Gourcerol et al,[80] 2007	12	29	5	1	69	33	21	10
Holzer et al,[79] 2007	35	29	2	1	—	—	—	—
Melenhorst et al,[76] 2007	36	33	10	2	79	59	—	—
Melenhorst et al,[76] 2007	48	15	10	2	—	—	—	—
Melenhorst et al,[76] 2007	60	10	10	2	—	—	—	—
Tjandra et al,[134] 2008	12	53	10	3	71	63	47	42
Munoz-Duyos et al,[135] 2008	36	29	1	0	86	58	48	33
El-Gazzaz et al,[136] 2009	28	24	5	2	—	—	—	—
Govaert et al,[137] 2009	35	169	—	—	77	53	—	—
Dudding et al,[138] 2009	51	18	6	0	94	—	39	—
Altomare et al,[139] 2009	74	52	4	1	—	—	18	10
Matzel et al,[84] 2009	118	9	9	0	78	58	44	33

Study								
Wexner et al,[82] 2010	12	106	9	1	83	66	—	—
Koch et al,[65] 2010	24	35	11	2	—	—	21	11
Michelsen et al,[140] 2010	24	126	8	1	—	—	—	—
Oom et al,[44] 2010	32	37	9	0	81	65	5	4
Ratto et al,[77] 2010	33	10	26	1	—	—	—	—
Lombardi et al,[141] 2010	46	11	5	1	100	—	27	—
Boyle et al,[75] 2011	17	37	7	1	73	54	46	40
Hollingshead et al,[142] 2011	33	86	9	1	83	—	—	—
Mellgren et al,[85] 2011	36	77	9	2	86	59	40	26
Uludağ et al,[71] 2011	85	50	8	0	84	—	—	—
Santoro et al,[143] 2012	18	16	14	0	—	—	68	68
Duelund-Jakobsen et al,[144] 2012	46	147	6	1	75	—	36	—
Devroede et al,[145] 2012	48	77	9	2	87	50	34	20
George et al,[97] 2012	114	23	9	2	—	—	52	48
Hull et al,[83] 2013	60	72	9	2	89	—	36	—

tenth that of SNS.[96–99] PTNS, however, requires repetitive treatments to maintain effectiveness. Weekly returns to the clinic for 12 consecutive weeks followed by maintenance visits may not be suitable for some patients. Thus, the success of PTNS depends highly on patients' motivation.

Until recently, the existing data on PTNS were derived from case series demonstrating that 52% to 83% achieved a greater than or equal to 50% reduction in frequency of FI.[96,100,101] The duration and frequency of the therapy vary, however, among the studies, making direct comparisons difficult. The largest prospective study, including 115 patients with a median follow-up of 26 months (range, 12–42), reported 52% of patients achieving a greater than or equal to 50% reduction in FI episodes as well as improving QOL.[100,102] The first multicenter RCT (Control of Faecal Incontinence using Distal Neuromoulation [CONFIDeNT]) in the United Kingdom was recently published. This trial included 227 patients to evaluate the efficacy and cost-effectiveness of PTNS (n = 115) compared with sham electrical stimulation (n = 112). The study reported no difference between the PTNS and sham groups in the efficacy at 12 weeks; 38% in PTNS versus 31% in sham have achieved a greater than or equal to 50% reduction in the number of FI episodes per week with the adjusted ratio of 1.28 (95% CI, 0.72–2.28; P = .40).[103]

Data comparing PTNS and SNS are limited. Al Asari and colleagues[98] reported no significant differences in the mean Wexner and Fecal Incontinence Quality of Life Scale (FIQoL) scores between PTNS and SNS groups up to 12 months on treatment of refractory FI. An RCT comparing PTNS and SNS in the treatment of FI is currently being undertaken in Switzerland (NCT01069016).[100,104]

Another form of PTNS is the transcutaneous approach using cutaneous pads instead of a needle.[105] This less-invasive device may allow patients to self-administer the treatment at home and potentially become a cost-effective option. Existing data on the efficacy of the transcutaneous approach are, however, limited. As more data become available, the ideal treatment protocol (interval, duration, and stimulation approach) as well as the role of PTNS for treatment of FI should be validated.

Perianal Injectables

Perianal injection of a bulking agent to increase the resting anal sphincter tone was first described in 1993.[106] Before the injectable therapy was available, the treatment of passive incontinence and IAS dysfunction was limited. Bulking materials into the submucosa or intersphincteric space increase the tissue volume in the high-pressure zone, especially in the proximal sphincter canal, creating a tighter seal at rest. Injectables could also target defective areas of the IAS, if present, to create canal symmetry.[107,108] Bulking agents introduced to date include autologous fat, Polytetra-fluoroethylene, bovine glutaraldehyde cross-linked collagen (Contigen), carbon-coated zirconium beads (Durasphere), polydimethylsiloxane elastomer, dextranomer in nonanimal stabilized hyaluronic acid, hydrogel cross-linked with polyacrylamide (Bioplastique), porcine dermal collagen (Permacol), synthetic calcium hydroxylapatite ceramic microspheres, and polyacrylonitrile in cylinder form. In 2011, nonanimal stabilized hyaluronic acid/dextranomer (NASHA/Dx) was approved by the FDA for the treatment of FI refractory to conservative therapy (**Fig. 2**). In the lithotomy, left-lateral, or prone position, 1 mL is injected into the deep submucosa through an ano-scope at 4 sites (typically, 3-o'clock, 6-o'clock, 9-o'clock, and 12-o'clock positions), slightly above the dentate line, targeting the proximal part of high pressure zone. When the response is not satisfactory, a repeat injection can be administered after 4 weeks. Given the minimally invasive technique, this therapy can be an office procedure with significantly low morbidity.

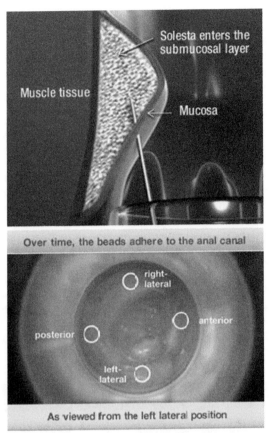

Fig. 2. Dextranomer-microspheres in sodium hyaluronate gel injection (Solesta). (*Courtesy of* Salix Pharmaceuticals, a division of Valeant Pharmaceuticals, Inc, Raleigh, NC; with permission.)

A double-blinded RCT for the short-term efficacy of NASHA/Dx versus sham injections for FI demonstrated that 52% in the NASHA/Dx group and 31% in the sham group achieved a greater than or equal to 50% reduction in FI episodes. At 12 months, the treatment response increased to 69% in the NASHA/Dx group. No difference was observed between the 2 groups at 3 months, suggesting the placebo effects cannot be negated.[106,108] The study was extended to 36 months evaluating the long-term efficacy. Of the 136 patients randomized to the NASHA/Dx group in the initial study, 82% (112/136) were available for the long-term assessment. The study showed that the success rate (a ≥50% reduction in FI episodes) was sustained at 52.2% at 36 months' follow-up. Complete continence was seen in 13.2% at 36 months, increased from 6% at 6 months. A majority of the patients (82% in the original study and 87% in the long-term follow-up study) received a second injection after 4 weeks from their initial treatment. No patients received further injections.[109] Common treatment-related adverse events were transient and minor bleeding, pain, and discomfort, mostly self-resolved. Of the 136 patients, only 2 had serious adverse events (abscesses) within 6 months, which were treated with antibiotics or surgical intervention. Adverse events unique to long-term follow-up (6–36 months) are injection site nodules seen in 2%.[106,108]

Although complete continence may not be achieved, perianal bulking therapy may be an effective and safe option to alleviate symptoms, especially in patients with mild to moderate passive FI. The evidence on NASHA/Dx is currently limited, however, to short-term efficacy. The injection techniques (submucosal vs intersphincteric space, transanal ultrasound guidance, and injection volume) and the optimal injectable substances are yet to be determined.

Radiofrequency Ablation Therapy

RF ablation therapy (Secca [Mederi Therapeutics Inc, Norwalk, CT]) was approved by the FDA in 2002 for treatment of refractory FI. This therapy device consists of an anoscope with 4 nickel-titanium curved needle electrodes to apply a temperature-controlled RF energy (65°C to 85°C) to the submucosa of the IAS (**Fig. 3**). In theory, heat applied to the submucosa induces collagen denaturation and tissue fibrosis; thus, the affected anal canal becomes constricted with increased resistance to stool passage.[110,111] A similar technique has been used for gastroesophageal reflux disease and benign prostatic hypertrophy.[110] The long-term (5-year) study of the Secca system reported that the mean Wexner Fecal Incontinence Score improved from 14 to 8 (*P*<.0003), and 84% of the subjects achieved greater than or equal to 50% symptomatic improvements. The study was limited, however, by a small sample size of only 19 patients.[112] Current data on the efficacy and safety of the Secca system are limited by the short-term follow-ups and small sample sizes because existing studies included neither greater than 50 patients (n = 8–50) nor follow-up longer than 5 years (6–60 months).[111–113] Therefore, there is insufficient evidence for the use of RF ablation.

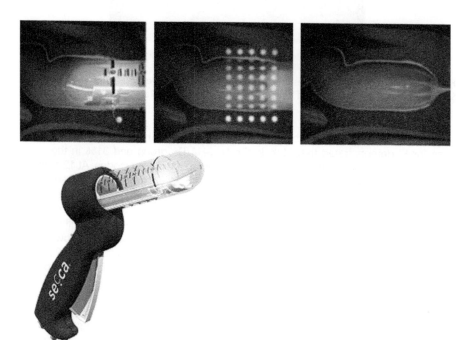

Fig. 3. RF ablation therapy (Secca). Secca is inserted in the anal canal, and temperature-controlled RF energy is delivered to the sphincter muscle (*above panels*). (*Copyright ©* 2015 Mederi Therapeutics Inc.)

Fecal Diversion

A colostomy or ileostomy is considered a definitive therapy yet the last option when other treatments have failed or are unsuitable. Many people are afraid that having an ostomy will have a greater negative impact on their QOL than living with FI. Early discussion regarding treatment options, including diversion, is helpful for coping with possible lifestyle changes in patients with severe FI, if appropriate. People with an ostomy can be active in their social and professional lives. Most activities, including sports, can be performed with minimal modifications. Ostomy should not affect sexual function. A study reported that both general QOL and disease-specific QOL were better in patients with colostomy; the colostomy group had higher scores on social function on the 36-Item Short Form Health Survey as well as the coping, embarrassment, lifestyle, and depression scales on the FIQoL compared with patients with FI.[114] Another study demonstrated that most patients with previous FI felt positively about having a stoma, with the median score of 8 for the ability to live with a stoma and 9 for satisfaction with the stoma (both on a scale of 0–10). The majority (83%) reported the stoma restricted their life "a little" or "not at all" with significant improvement from their previous incontinence.[115] Fecal diversion via laparoscopy is a safe and effective option with decreased morbidity, such as reduced postoperative pain, ileus, and the length of hospital stay.[11,116,117] Although considered a last resort, diverting ostomy can ameliorate symptoms and improve QOL in women with severe refractory FI.

Recently Available Treatment Options: Devices

Anal plugs

Anal plugs are designed to temporarily occlude the anal canal to prevent stool leakage.

Existing studies suggest that anal plugs may be difficult to tolerate, as demonstrated by a considerably high dropout rate (35%). If tolerated, the device may be helpful to alleviate symptoms, particularly in patients with impaired anal-rectal sensation and those who are institutionalized or immobilized.[118] The REST study is the most recent multicenter, prospective, single-arm, nonrandomized trial to evaluate the safety, tolerability, and effectiveness of a new single-use disposable device (the Renew Insert, Renew Medical, Inc, Foster City, CA), including 91 patients with moderate-to-severe FI.[119] The device is a silicone anal insert, designed for self-insertion, with an applicator to seal the rectum to help prevent leakage and is naturally expelled with a bowel movement (**Fig. 4**). Of the 91 subjects (ITT cohort), 73 (80%) completed all 12 weeks of treatment (completers), whereas 85 (93%) completed at least 1 week of treatment (modified ITT [mITT] cohort). The study showed a significant reduction in FI frequency, 0.9 FI episodes per day at baseline to 0.2 episodes at 12 weeks ($P<0.001$) in the mITT cohort. A greater than or equal to 50% reduction in FI frequency was seen in 62% and 78% of the ITT and mITT cohorts, respectively. The study also demonstrated a significant reduction in the Wexner scores (16.2 baseline vs 10.9 with treatment, $P<0.001$). Adverse events were seen in 51%; however, almost all (98%) events were mild, such as anorectal urgency (26%), irritation (13%), gastrointestinal discomfort (4%), gas (3%), or hemorrhoids (6%). Subjectively, 78% of the completers were either very or extremely satisfied with the device.[119]

Vaginal bowel control system

A vaginal bowel control system (Eclipse System [Pelvalon, Inc, Sunnyvale, CA]) has been designed to provide a low-risk, effective, and easily reversible treatment for women with FI. The device consists of a silicone-coated base with an inflatable balloon and a handheld pressure-regulated pump. The system is inserted into the

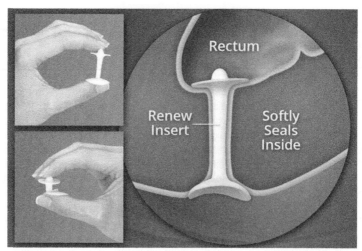

Fig. 4. Anal plug (RENEW Inserts). (*Reprinted* with permission of Renew Medical, Inc.)

vagina, similar to a pessary, with the balloon directed posteriorly. When the balloon is inflated, the vaginal wall occupies rectal space, preventing unwanted stool passage. Deflating the balloon allows stool passage; thus, patients are able to control their own bowel movements (**Fig. 5**). Typically, the vaginal insertion produces little or no sensation. The LIFE (LivSure for Fecal Incontinence) study was a trial for women with FI to evaluate the effectiveness and safely of the Eclipse device. Of 110 subjects,

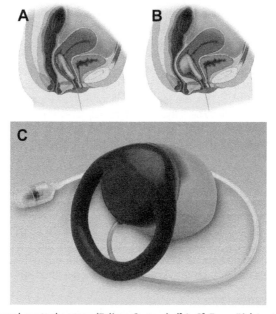

Fig. 5. Vaginal bowel control system (Eclipse System). ([*A, B*] *From* Richter HE, Matthews CA, Takase-Sanchez MM, et al. A vaginal bowel-control system for the treatment of fecal incontinence. Obstet Gynecol 2015;125(3):541. Wolters Kluwer Health, Inc; with permission; and [*C*] *Courtesy of* Pelvalon, Inc; with permission.)

61 were successfully fitted with the device and subsequently proceeded with a 4-week treatment period. The study reported 79% (ITT) and 86% (per protocol) reported a greater than or equal to 50% reduction in FI episodes. Subjectively, 86% reported their bowel symptoms "very much better" or "much better," and a significant improvement in QOL was demonstrated using the FIQoL and Modified Manchester Health Questionnaire subscales. Adverse events were observed in 47 of 110 participants (all mild to moderate), and many device-related events were noted during the fitting period, including 15% pelvic discomfort, 10% urinary leakage or urgency, 9% vaginal findings (erythema, abrasions, and irritation), 8% pelvic pain, and 7% vaginal spotting. During the treatment period, the rate of adverse events were much lower, with 10% pelvic discomfort, 3% urinary incontinence or urgency, 5% vaginal findings, and 3% pelvic pain.[120] Currently, the device is being investigated on the durability of the safety and effectiveness for extended follow-up periods (3 and 12 months of use) by a multicenter, prospective, open-label clinical trial (LIBERATE study, A Clinical Evaluation of the Eclipse System, a Vaginal Bowel Control Therapy for Fecal Incontinence in Women, NCT02428595).

Investigational Treatment Options

Autologous myoblast injection

Autologous myoblast injection is an investigational procedure. Because the anal sphincter muscles degenerate over time on injury, leading to sphincter dysfunction, injection of autologous cells can potentially replace or repair the damaged tissue and enhance their function. The exact mechanisms and histomorphologic and functional changes of disrupted sphincter muscles in response to myoblasts are being studied using animal models.[121–123] In humans, similar regenerative therapy with autologous cells injected into the urethral sphincter in patients with stress urinary incontinence seems beneficial in small investigational studies.[124,125] The pilot study has been conducted to evaluate the clinical efficacy of the autologous myoblast cell injection (cultured and harvested from the pectoralis muscle) in women with symptomatic FI due to disrupted EAS from obstetric trauma. This study demonstrated an increase in squeeze pressures at 1 and 6 months postinjection; however, they returned to baseline by 12 months. In addition, significant improvements were noted in both overall symptoms and QOL as measured by the Wexner score and FIQoL scale at 12 months postinjection.[126] An RCT of intrasphincteric injections with autologous myoblasts versus saline solution is being undertaken (NCT01523522). Autologous cells have definite advantages over embryonic stem cells because the former avoids adverse events related to foreign materials and bypass ethical concerns.

Magnetic anal sphincter

Anal sphincter augmentation using a magnetic ring has been introduced to treat FI. The FENIX Continence Restoration System (Torax Medical, Inc, Shoreview, MN) consists of a flexible band of interlinked titanium beads, each with a magnetic core, to form a ring. The magnetic attractions among the beads reinforce the closing pressure of the anal sphincter to prevent leakage of stool. Straining to defecate separates the beads to allow voluntary passage of stool (**Fig. 6**). This device is surgically implanted around the anal canal.[127,128] A similar device has been used to treat gastroesophageal reflux disease. Short-term to midterm efficacy of seems promising.[127,129,130] One study with a median follow-up of 18 (6–45) months reported a success rate of 70% (defined as improvement of the postoperative Cleveland Clinic Florida Incontinence Severity [CCF-IS] score by >50%). In the same study, the QOL scores (measured by the FIQoL) also improved postoperatively.[127] Another prospective study reported improved QOL

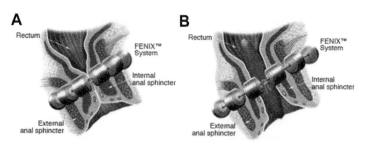

Fig. 6. Magnetic anal sphincter (FENIX Continence Restoration System). (*A*) Magnetic attraction augmenting the anal sphincter. (*B*) Magnetic anal sphincter expands to allow passage of stool. (*Reprinted* with permission of Torax Medical, Inc.)

and decreased incontinence severity (measured by the FIQoL and CCF-FIS scores, respectively) and demonstrated 76% of the subjects having greater than or equal to 50% reduction in FI episodes per week.[131] Current data, however, are derived from observational studies with a small sample size (7–23 subjects).[127,129–131] In addition, the definition of success varies among the studies, making direct comparisons difficult. A randomized trial with a larger sample size is needed to further evaluate the long-term efficacy and safety of magnetic anal sphincter.

Sling for fecal incontinence

The Trans-Obturator Post-Anal Sling (TOPAS, American Medical Systems, Minnetonka, MN) system is a self-fixating polypropylene mesh placed under the anorectum to provide anatomic support. The mesh is placed lateral to the puborectalis muscle and inferior to the anorectum and brought through the ischiorectal fossa using 2 needle passers via the transobturator approach, thus reinforcing the normal anorectal angle. A prospective multicenter open-label study, including 29 women, reported a significant decrease in the mean number of FI episodes per 14 days (from 6.9 to 3.5 episodes) at 24 months. In addition, 56% of the subjects reported treatment success, defined as a greater than or equal to 50% reduction in number of FI episodes per 14 days compared with baseline. Device-related adverse events were observed in 12 patients, with total 19 events during the study period. The most common events were de novo urinary incontinence or bladder spasm (n = 6), worsening FI (n = 2), and constipation (n = 2), and 1 patient had disk herniation related to the positioning during the procedure. No device erosions or extrusions were noted in the 24-month follow-up period.[132]

There is an ongoing prospective multicenter, single-arm open label study (15 colorectal surgery and urogynecology centers in the United States). The TRANSFORM (Treatment of Fecal Incontinence using the TOPAS Sling System for Women, NCT01090739) study is evaluating the safety and effectiveness of the TOPAS system for the treatment of FI in women who failed conservative therapy. The study included 152 women with FI who were implanted with the TOPAS system. Treatment success was defined as a greater than or equal to 50% reduction in number of FI episodes. Outcomes were assessed at baseline, 3 months, 6 months, and 12 months postoperatively. Preliminary results showed that 69% of women had a greater than or equal to 50% reduction in FI episodes. The median frequency was 9 episodes and 5 incontinence days per week at baseline down to 2.5 episodes and 2 incontinence days per week at 12 months. Treatment-related adverse events were seen in 71 patients with a total of 113 events; 97% were managed without therapy or through nonsurgical treatment. The most common complications (>5%) were pain, primarily in the buttock, pelvis, or groin, and incision site infection. No mesh erosions, extrusions, organ per-forations, bowel obstructions, or device revisions were reported.[133] The final report has yet to be published.

SUMMARY/DISCUSSION

FI is a physically and psychosocially debilitating disorder that has a negative impact on QOL. Despite a reasonably high prevalence rate, many women are reluctant to report symptoms and seek care and thus feel succumbed to the condition. In addition, health care providers often fail to screen for FI not only due to the complexity in evaluation but also because of the limited awareness of the prevalence and lack of clinical experi-ence and knowledge on currently available therapies.

Treatment of FI can be challenging because the etiology is often multifactorial. Pre-vention and early intervention should focus on eliminating potential modifiable risk factors, such as loose stool, diarrhea, routine practice of episiotomy, and operative vaginal delivery, especially forceps assisted, and identifying women suffering from FI at earlier stages to avoid worsening symptoms. Management consists of conserva-tive and surgical approaches, and more-invasive therapies are reserved for patients with refractory conditions. Traditionally, treatment options were limited once patients failed conservative therapies. Surgery for FI was considered invasive with high complication rates, and the success rates deteriorated over time. Recent research, however, has provided additional data on the existing treatments as well as the devel-opment of less-invasive options and new investigational treatments. Of the currently available options, only 3 therapy modalities have been evaluated by RCTs with suffi-cient size to provide level I evidence, which include biofeedback, NASHA/Dx perianal injection, and PTNS. Although SNS is supported by strong level II evidence, the cur-rent RCT data on SNS are derived from patients with intact EAS and FI without neuro-logic disorders; thus, generalizability is limited. Based on the US Preventative Services Task Force scoring system, most treatments were assigned grade B recom-mendations. Biofeedback is the only modality with a grade A recommendation.[93] Further RCTs evaluating long-term efficacy and safety of each modality as well as well-designed comparative studies of available options and the effectiveness of com-bination therapies are still needed to solidify a management algorithm for FI. In addi-tion, future research should focus on the cost effectiveness of current therapies because direct and indirect costs associated with FI are substantial. The optimal treatment regimen is often a combination of various conservative and surgical approaches. As more data emerge, health care providers should become familiar with the available options and critically evaluate both immediate and long-term out-comes on the efficacy and safety and individualize FI management using evidence-based practice.

REFERENCES

1. Wald A. Clinical practice. Fecal incontinence in adults. N Engl J Med 2007;356: 1648–55.
2. Markland AD, Richter HE, Burgio KL, et al. Weight loss improves fecal inconti-nence severity in overweight and obese women with urinary incontinence. Int Urogynecol J 2011;22:1151–7.
3. Nygaard I, Barber MD, Burgio KL, et al. Prevalence of symptomatic pelvic floor disorders in US women. JAMA 2008;300:1311–6.

4. Lawrence JM, Lukacz ES, Nager CW, et al. Prevalence and co-occurrence of pelvic floor disorders in community-dwelling women. Obstet Gynecol 2008; 111:678–85.
5. Gleason JL, Markland A, Greer WJ, et al. Anal sphincter repair for fecal incontinence: effect on symptom severity, quality of life, and anal sphincter squeeze pressures. Int Urogynecol J 2011;22:1587–92.
6. Varma MG, Brown JS, Creasman JM, et al, Reproductive Risks for Incontinence Study at Kaiser Research Group. Fecal incontinence in females older than aged 40 years: who is at risk? Dis Colon Rectum 2006;49:841–51.
7. Markland AD, Goode PS, Burgio KL, et al. Incidence and risk factors for fecal incontinence in black and white older adults: a population-based study. J Am Geriatr Soc 2010;58:1341–6.
8. Kang HW, Jung HK, Kwon KJ, et al. Prevalence and predictive factors of fecal incontinence. J Neurogastroenterol Motil 2012;18:86–93.
9. Dunivan GC, Heymen S, Palsson OS, et al. Fecal incontinence in primary care: prevalence, diagnosis, and health care utilization. Am J Obstet Gynecol 2010; 202(493):e491–496.
10. Johanson JF, Lafferty J. Epidemiology of fecal incontinence: the silent affliction. Am J Gastroenterol 1996;91:33–6.
11. Rao SS, American College of Gastroenterology Practice Parameters Committee. Diagnosis and management of fecal incontinence. American College of Gastroenterology Practice Parameters Committee. Am J Gastroenterol 2004; 99:1585–604.
12. Degen LP, Phillips SF. How well does stool form reflect colonic transit? Gut 1996; 39:109–13.
13. Saad RJ, Rao SS, Koch KL, et al. Do stool form and frequency correlate with whole-gut and colonic transit? Results from a multicenter study in constipated individuals and healthy controls. Am J Gastroenterol 2010;105:403–11.
14. Bliss DZ, Savik K, Jung HJ, et al. Dietary fiber supplementation for fecal incontinence: a randomized clinical trial. Res Nurs Health 2014;37:367–78.
15. Eswaran S, Muir J, Chey WD. Fiber and functional gastrointestinal disorders. Am J Gastroenterol 2013;108:718–27.
16. Wang JY, Abbas MA. Current management of fecal incontinence. Perm J 2013; 17:65–73.
17. Ehrenpreis ED, Chang D, Eichenwald E. Pharmacotherapy for fecal incontinence: a review. Dis Colon Rectum 2007;50:641–9.
18. Read M, Read NW, Barber DC, et al. Effects of loperamide on anal sphincter function in patients complaining of chronic diarrhea with fecal incontinence and urgency. Dig Dis Sci 1982;27:807–14.
19. Omar MI, Alexander CE. Drug treatment for faecal incontinence in adults. Cochrane Database Syst Rev 2013;(6):CD002116.
20. Palmer KR, Corbett CL, Holdsworth CD. Double-blind cross-over study comparing loperamide, codeine and diphenoxylate in the treatment of chronic diarrhea. Gastroenterology 1980;79:1272–5.
21. Markland AD, Burgio KL, Whitehead WE, et al. Loperamide versus psyllium fiber for treatment of fecal incontinence: the fecal incontinence prescription (Rx) management (FIRM) randomized clinical trial. Dis Colon Rectum 2015; 58:983–93.
22. Eric Jelovsek J, Markland AD, Whitehead WE, et al. Controlling anal incontinence in women by performing anal exercises with biofeedback or loperamide (CAPABLe) trial: design and methods. Contemp Clin Trials 2015;44:164–74.

23. Costilla VC, Foxx-Orenstein AE, Mayer AP, et al. Office-based management of fecal incontinence. Gastroenterol Hepatol 2013;9:423–33.
24. Remes-Troche JM, Ozturk R, Philips C, et al. Cholestyramine–a useful adjunct for the treatment of patients with fecal incontinence. Int J Colorectal Dis 2008; 23:189–94.
25. Trinkley KE, Nahata MC. Medication management of irritable bowel syndrome. Digestion 2014;89:253–67.
26. Bharucha AE, Fletcher JG, Camilleri M, et al. Effects of clonidine in women with fecal incontinence. Clin Gastroenterol Hepatol 2014;12:843–51.
27. Cheetham MJ, Kamm MA, Phillips RK. Topical phenylephrine increases anal canal resting pressure in patients with faecal incontinence. Gut 2001;48: 356–9.
28. Byrne CM, Solomon MJ, Young JM, et al. Biofeedback for fecal incontinence: short-term outcomes of 513 consecutive patients and predictors of successful treatment. Dis Colon Rectum 2007;50:417–27.
29. Norton C, Cody JD. Biofeedback and/or sphincter exercises for the treatment of faecal incontinence in adults. Cochrane Database Syst Rev 2012;(7):CD002111.
30. Madoff RD, Parker SC, Varma MG, et al. Faecal incontinence in adults. Lancet 2004;364:621–32.
31. Norton C, Chelvanayagam S, Wilson-Barnett J, et al. Randomized controlled trial of biofeedback for fecal incontinence. Gastroenterology 2003;125:1320–9.
32. Heymen S, Scarlett Y, Jones K, et al. Randomized controlled trial shows biofeedback to be superior to pelvic floor exercises for fecal incontinence. Dis Colon Rectum 2009;52:1730–7.
33. Solomon MJ, Pager CK, Rex J, et al. Randomized, controlled trial of biofeedback with anal manometry, transanal ultrasound, or pelvic floor retraining with digital guidance alone in the treatment of mild to moderate fecal incontinence. Dis Colon Rectum 2003;46:703–10.
34. Landefeld CS, Bowers BJ, Feld AD, et al. National Institutes of Health state-of-the-science conference statement: prevention of fecal and urinary incontinence in adults. Ann Intern Med 2008;148:449–58.
35. Anandam JL. Surgical management for fecal incontinence. Clin Colon Rectal Surg 2014;27:106–9.
36. Bradley CS, Richter HE, Gutman RE, et al, Pelvic Floor Disorders Network. Risk factors for sonographic internal anal sphincter gaps 6-12 months after delivery complicated by anal sphincter tear. Am J Obstet Gynecol 2007;197:310.e1–5.
37. Parks AG, McPartlin JF. Late repair of injuries of the anal sphincter. Proc R Soc Med 1971;64:1187–9.
38. Fang DT, Nivatvongs S, Vermeulen FD, et al. Overlapping sphincteroplasty for acquired anal incontinence. Dis Colon Rectum 1984;27:720–2.
39. Oberwalder M, Dinnewitzer A, Baig MK, et al. Do internal anal sphincter defects decrease the success rate of anal sphincter repair? Tech Coloproctol 2006;10: 94–7 [discussion: 97].
40. Wexner SD, Marchetti F, Jagelman DG. The role of sphincteroplasty for fecal incontinence reevaluated: a prospective physiologic and functional review. Dis Colon Rectum 1991;34:22–30.
41. Aitola P, Hiltunen KM, Matikainen M. Functional results of anterior levatorplasty and external sphincter plication for faecal incontinence. Ann Chir Gynaecol 2000;89:29–32.
42. Mellgren A, Anzén B, Nilsson BY, et al. Results of rectocele repair. A prospective study. Dis Colon Rectum 1995;38:7–13.

43. Kahn MA, Stanton SL. Posterior colporrhaphy: its effects on bowel and sexual function. Br J Obstet Gynaecol 1997;104:82–6.
44. Oom DM, Steensma AB, van Lanschot JJ, et al. Is sacral neuromodulation for fecal incontinence worthwhile in patients with associated pelvic floor injury? Dis Colon Rectum 2010;53:422–7.
45. Sung VW, Rogers ML, Myers DL, et al. National trends and costs of surgical treatment for female fecal incontinence. Am J Obstet Gynecol 2007;197: 652.e1–5.
46. Tjandra JJ, Han WR, Goh J, et al. Direct repair vs. overlapping sphincter repair: a randomized, controlled trial. Dis Colon Rectum 2003;46:937–42 [discussion: 942–3].
47. Garcia V, Rogers RG, Kim SS, et al. Primary repair of obstetric anal sphincter laceration: a randomized trial of two surgical techniques. Am J Obstet Gynecol 2005;192:1697–701.
48. Bravo Gutierrez A, Madoff RD, Lowry AC, et al. Long-term results of anterior sphincteroplasty. Dis Colon Rectum 2004;47:727–31 [discussion: 731–2].
49. Glasgow SC, Lowry AC. Long-term outcomes of anal sphincter repair for fecal incontinence: a systematic review. Dis Colon Rectum 2012;55:482–90.
50. Sultan AH, Kamm MA, Hudson CN, et al. Anal-sphincter disruption during vaginal delivery. N Engl J Med 1993;329:1905–11.
51. Bharucha AE, Fletcher JG, Harper CM, et al. Relationship between symptoms and disordered continence mechanisms in women with idiopathic faecal incontinence. Gut 2005;54:546–55.
52. MacArthur C, Glazener C, Lancashire R, et al, ProLong Study Group. Exclusive caesarean section delivery and subsequent urinary and faecal incontinence: a 12-year longitudinal study. BJOG 2011;118:1001–7.
53. Pretlove SJ, Thompson PJ, Toozs-Hobson PM, et al. Does the mode of delivery predispose women to anal incontinence in the first year postpartum? A comparative systematic review. BJOG 2008;115:421–34.
54. Handa VL, Blomquist JL, Knoepp LR, et al. Pelvic floor disorders 5-10 years after vaginal or cesarean childbirth. Obstet Gynecol 2011;118:777–84.
55. Nelson RL, Furner SE, Westercamp M, et al. Cesarean delivery for the prevention of anal incontinence. Cochrane Database Syst Rev 2010;(2):CD006756.
56. Nager CW, Helliwell JP. Episiotomy increases perineal laceration length in primiparous women. Am J Obstet Gynecol 2001;185:444–50.
57. Boggs EW, Berger H, Urquia M, et al. Recurrence of obstetric third-degree and fourth-degree anal sphincter injuries. Obstet Gynecol 2014;124:1128–34.
58. Edozien LC, Gurol-Urganci I, Cromwell DA, et al. Impact of third- and fourth-degree perineal tears at first birth on subsequent pregnancy outcomes: a cohort study. BJOG 2014;121:1695–703.
59. American College of Obstetricians and Gynecologists. ACOG committee opinion no. 559: Cesarean delivery on maternal request. Obstet Gynecol 2013;121: 904–7.
60. Elfaghi I, Johansson-Ernste B, Rydhstroem H. Rupture of the sphincter ani: the recurrence rate in second delivery. BJOG 2004;111:1361–4.
61. McKenna DS, Ester JB, Fischer JR. Elective cesarean delivery for women with a previous anal sphincter rupture. Am J Obstet Gynecol 2003;189:1251–6.
62. Farrell SA, Flowerdew G, Gilmour D, et al. Overlapping compared with end-to-end repair of complete third-degree or fourth-degree obstetric tears: three-year follow-up of a randomized controlled trial. Obstet Gynecol 2012;120: 803–8.

63. Khaikin M, Wexner SD. Treatment strategies in obstructed defecation and fecal incontinence. World J Gastroenterol 2006;12:3168–73.

64. Chapman AE, Geerdes B, Hewett P, et al. Systematic review of dynamic graciloplasty in the treatment of faecal incontinence. Br J Surg 2002;89: 138–53.

65. Koch SM, Melenhorst J, Uludağ O, et al. Sacral nerve modulation and other treatments in patients with faecal incontinence after unsuccessful pelvic floor rehabilitation: a prospective study. Colorectal Dis 2010;12:334–41.

66. Wong MT, Meurette G, Wyart V, et al. The artificial bowel sphincter: a single institution experience over a decade. Ann Surg 2011;254:951–6.

67. Mundy L, Merlin TL, Maddern GJ, et al. Systematic review of safety and effectiveness of an artificial bowel sphincter for faecal incontinence. Br J Surg 2004;91:665–72.

68. Hong KD, Dasilva G, Kalaskar SN, et al. Long-term outcomes of artificial bowel sphincter for fecal incontinence: a systematic review and meta-analysis. J Am Coll Surg 2013;217:718–25.

69. Matzel KE. Sacral nerve stimulation for faecal incontinence: its role in the treatment algorithm. Colorectal Dis 2011;13(Suppl 2):10–4.

70. Patton V, Wiklendt L, Arkwright JW, et al. The effect of sacral nerve stimulation on distal colonic motility in patients with faecal incontinence. Br J Surg 2013;100: 959–68.

71. Uludağ O, Melenhorst J, Koch SM, et al. Sacral neuromodulation: long-term outcome and quality of life in patients with faecal incontinence. Colorectal Dis 2011;13:1162–6.

72. Kenefick NJ, Vaizey CJ, Cohen RC, et al. Medium-term results of permanent sacral nerve stimulation for faecal incontinence. Br J Surg 2002;89:896–901.

73. Vaizey CJ, Kamm MA, Turner IC, et al. Effects of short term sacral nerve stimulation on anal and rectal function in patients with anal incontinence. Gut 1999;44: 407–12.

74. Rasmussen OO, Buntzen S, Sørensen M, et al. Sacral nerve stimulation in fecal incontinence. Dis Colon Rectum 2004;47:1158–62 [discussion: 1162–3].

75. Boyle DJ, Murphy J, Gooneratne ML, et al. Efficacy of sacral nerve stimulation for the treatment of fecal incontinence. Dis Colon Rectum 2011;54:1271–8.

76. Melenhorst J, Koch SM, Uludag O, et al. Sacral neuromodulation in patients with faecal incontinence: results of the first 100 permanent implantations. Colorectal Dis 2007;9:725–30.

77. Ratto C, Litta F, Parello A, et al. Sacral nerve stimulation is a valid approach in fecal incontinence due to sphincter lesions when compared to sphincter repair. Dis Colon Rectum 2010;53:264–72.

78. Jarrett ME, Dudding TC, Nicholls RJ, et al. Sacral nerve stimulation for fecal incontinence related to obstetric anal sphincter damage. Dis Colon Rectum 2008; 51:531–7.

79. Holzer B, Rosen HR, Novi G, et al. Sacral nerve stimulation for neurogenic faecal incontinence. Br J Surg 2007;94:749–53.

80. Gourcerol G, Gallas S, Michot F, et al. Sacral nerve stimulation in fecal incontinence: are there factors associated with success? Dis Colon Rectum 2007;50:3–12.

81. Baxter C, Kim JH. Contrasting the percutaneous nerve evaluation versus staged implantation in sacral neuromodulation. Curr Urol Rep 2010;11:310–4.

82. Wexner SD, Coller JA, Devroede G, et al. Sacral nerve stimulation for fecal incontinence: results of a 120-patient prospective multicenter study. Ann Surg 2010;251:441–9.

83. Hull T, Giese C, Wexner SD, et al. Long-term durability of sacral nerve stimulation therapy for chronic fecal incontinence. Dis Colon Rectum 2013;56: 234–45.

84. Matzel KE, Lux P, Heuer S, et al. Sacral nerve stimulation for faecal incontinence: long-term outcome. Colorectal Dis 2009;11:636–41.

85. Mellgren A, Wexner SD, Coller JA, et al. Long-term efficacy and safety of sacral nerve stimulation for fecal incontinence. Dis Colon Rectum 2011;54:1065–75.

86. Tan E, Ngo NT, Darzi A, et al. Meta-analysis: sacral nerve stimulation versus conservative therapy in the treatment of faecal incontinence. Int J Colorectal Dis 2011;26:275–94.

87. Tjandra JJ, Lim JF, Matzel K. Sacral nerve stimulation: an emerging treatment for faecal incontinence. ANZ J Surg 2004;74:1098–106.

88. Matzel KE, Kamm MA, Stosser M, et al. Sacral spinal nerve stimulation for faecal incontinence: multicentre study. Lancet 2004;363:1270–6.

89. Chiarioni G, Palsson OS, Asteria CR, et al. Neuromodulation for fecal incontinence: an effective surgical intervention. World J Gastroenterol 2013;19:7048–54.

90. Tan EK, Vaizey C, Cornish J, et al. Surgical strategies for faecal incontinence–a decision analysis between dynamic graciloplasty, artificial bowel sphincter and end stoma. Colorectal Dis 2008;10:577–86.

91. Wong MT, Meurette G, Rodat F, et al. Outcome and management of patients in whom sacral nerve stimulation for fecal incontinence failed. Dis Colon Rectum 2011;54:425–32.

92. Brown SR, Nelson RL. Surgery for faecal incontinence in adults. Cochrane Database Syst Rev 2007;(2):CD001757.

93. Whitehead WE, Rao SS, Lowry A, et al. Treatment of fecal incontinence: state of the science summary for the national institute of diabetes and digestive and kidney diseases workshop. Am J Gastroenterol 2015;110:138–46.

94. Wiseman OJ, v d Hombergh U, Koldewijn EL, et al. Sacral neuromodulation and pregnancy. J Urol 2002;167:165–8.

95. Khunda A, Karmarkar R, Abtahi B, et al. Pregnancy in women with Fowler's syndrome treated with sacral neuromodulation. Int Urogynecol J 2013;24:1201–4.

96. Thin NN, Horrocks EJ, Hotouras A, et al. Systematic review of the clinical effectiveness of neuromodulation in the treatment of faecal incontinence. Br J Surg 2013;100:1430–47.

97. George AT, Kalmar K, Panarese A, et al. Long-term outcomes of sacral nerve stimulation for fecal incontinence. Dis Colon Rectum 2012;55:302–6.

98. Al Asari S, Meurette G, Mantoo S, et al. Percutaneous tibial nerve stimulation vs sacral nerve stimulation for faecal incontinence: a comparative case-matched study. Colorectal Dis 2014;16:O393–9.

99. Klingler HC, Pycha A, Schmidbauer J, et al. Use of peripheral neuromodulation of the S3 region for treatment of detrusor overactivity: a urodynamic-based study. Urology 2000;56:766–71.

100. Hotouras A, Murphy J, Walsh U, et al. Outcome of percutaneous tibial nerve stimulation (PTNS) for fecal incontinence: a prospective cohort study. Ann Surg 2014;259:939–43.

101. Thomas GP, Dudding TC, Rahbour G, et al. A review of posterior tibial nerve stimulation for faecal incontinence. Colorectal Dis 2013;15:519–26.

102. Hotouras A, Murphy J, Allison M, et al. Prospective clinical audit of two neuromodulatory treatments for fecal incontinence: sacral nerve stimulation (SNS) and percutaneous tibial nerve stimulation (PTNS). Surg Today 2014;44(11): 2124–30.

103. Knowles CH, Horrocks EJ, Bremner SA, et al, CONFIDeNT Study Group. Percutaneous tibial nerve stimulation versus sham electrical stimulation for the treatment of faecal incontinence in adults (CONFIDeNT): a double-blind, multicentre, pragmatic, parallel-group, randomised controlled trial. Lancet 2015;386(10004):1640–8.
104. Lowman JK, Jones LA, Woodman PJ, et al. Does the Prolift system cause dyspareunia? Am J Obstet Gynecol 2008;199:707.e1–6.
105. Queralto M, Portier G, Cabarrot PH, et al. Preliminary results of peripheral transcutaneous neuromodulation in the treatment of idiopathic fecal incontinence. Int J Colorectal Dis 2006;21:670–2.
106. Graf W, Mellgren A, Matzel KE, et al. Efficacy of dextranomer in stabilised hyaluronic acid for treatment of faecal incontinence: a randomised, sham-controlled trial. Lancet 2011;377:997–1003.
107. Watson NF, Koshy A, Sagar PM. Anal bulking agents for faecal incontinence. Colorectal Dis 2012;14(Suppl 3):29–33.
108. Maeda Y, Laurberg S, Norton C. Perianal injectable bulking agents as treatment for faecal incontinence in adults. Cochrane Database Syst Rev 2013;(2):CD007959.
109. Mellgren A, Matzel KE, Pollack J, et al. Long-term efficacy of NASHA Dx injection therapy for treatment of fecal incontinence. Neurogastroenterol Motil 2014; 26(8):1087–94.
110. Parisien CJ, Corman ML. The Secca procedure for the treatment of fecal incontinence: definitive therapy or short-term solution. Clin Colon Rectal Surg 2005; 18:42–5.
111. Frascio M, Mandolfino F, Imperatore M, et al. The SECCA procedure for faecal incontinence: a review. Colorectal Dis 2014;16:167–72.
112. Takahashi-Monroy T, Morales M, Garcia-Osogobio S, et al. SECCA procedure for the treatment of fecal incontinence: results of five-year follow-up. Dis Colon Rectum 2008;51:355–9.
113. The National Institute for Health and Clinical Excellence. Endoscopic radiofrequency therapy of the anal sphincter for faecal incontinence. London: Interventional Procedure Guidance; 2011.
114. Colquhoun P, Kaiser R, Efron J, et al. Is the quality of life better in patients with colostomy than patients with fecal incontience? World J Surg 2006;30:1925–8.
115. Norton C, Burch J, Kamm MA. Patients' views of a colostomy for fecal incontinence. Dis Colon Rectum 2005;48:1062–9.
116. Ludwig KA, Milsom JW, Garcia-Ruiz A, et al. Laparoscopic techniques for fecal diversion. Dis Colon Rectum 1996;39:285–8.
117. Lyerly HK, Mault JR. Laparoscopic ileostomy and colostomy. Ann Surg 1994; 219:317–22.
118. Deutekom M, Dobben AC. Plugs for containing faecal incontinence. Cochrane Database Syst Rev 2015;(7):CD005086.
119. Lukacz ES, Segall MM, Wexner SD. Evaluation of an anal insert device for the conservative management of fecal incontinence. Dis Colon Rectum 2015;58:892–8.
120. Richter HE, Matthews CA, Muir T, et al. A vaginal bowel-control system for the treatment of fecal incontinence. Obstet Gynecol 2015;125:540–7.
121. Lane FL, Jacobs SA, Craig JB, et al. In vivo recovery of the injured anal sphincter after repair and injection of myogenic stem cells: an experimental model. Dis Colon Rectum 2013;56:1290–7.
122. Fitzwater JL, Grande KB, Sailors JL, et al. Effect of myogenic stem cells on the integrity and histomorphology of repaired transected external anal sphincter. Int Urogynecol J 2015;26:251–6.

123. Montoya TI, Acevedo JF, Smith B, et al. Myogenic stem cell-laden hydrogel scaffold in wound healing of the disrupted external anal sphincter. Int Urogynecol J 2015;26(6):893–904.
124. Carr LK, Robert M, Kultgen PL, et al. Autologous muscle derived cell therapy for stress urinary incontinence: a prospective, dose ranging study. J Urol 2013;189: 595–601.
125. Carr LK, Steele D, Steele S, et al. 1-year follow-up of autologous muscle-derived stem cell injection pilot study to treat stress urinary incontinence. Int Urogynecol J Pelvic Floor Dysfunct 2008;19:881–3.
126. Frudinger A, Kölle D, Schwaiger W, et al. Muscle-derived cell injection to treat anal incontinence due to obstetric trauma: pilot study with 1 year follow-up. Gut 2010;59:55–61.
127. Barussaud ML, Mantoo S, Wyart V, et al. The magnetic anal sphincter in faecal incontinence: is initial success sustained over time? Colorectal Dis 2013;15: 1499–503.
128. Mantoo S, Meurette G, Podevin J, et al. The magnetic anal sphincter: a new device in the management of severe fecal incontinence. Expert Rev Med Devices 2012;9:483–90.
129. Wong MT, Meurette G, Wyart V, et al. Does the magnetic anal sphincter device compare favourably with sacral nerve stimulation in the management of faecal incontinence? Colorectal Dis 2012;14:e323–329.
130. Wong MT, Meurette G, Stangherlin P, et al. The magnetic anal sphincter versus the artificial bowel sphincter: a comparison of 2 treatments for fecal incontinence. Dis Colon Rectum 2011;54:773–9.
131. Pakravan F, Helmes C. Magnetic anal sphincter augmentation in patients with severe fecal incontinence. Dis Colon Rectum 2015;58:109–14.
132. Rosenblatt P, Schumacher J, Lucente V, et al. A preliminary evaluation of the TOPAS system for the treatment of fecal incontinence in women. Female Pelvic Med Reconstr Surg 2014;20:155–62.
133. Fenner D, Lucente V, Zutshi M, et al. TOPASTM System. A New Modality for the Treatment of Fecal Incontinence in Women. J Minim Invasive Gynecol 2015;22: S3–4.
134. Tjandra JJ, Chan MK, Yeh CH, et al. Sacral nerve stimulation is more effective than optimal medical therapy for severe fecal incontinence: a randomized, controlled study. Dis Colon Rectum 2008;51:494–502.
135. Munoz-Duyos A, Navarro-Luna A, Brosa M, et al. Clinical and cost effectiveness of sacral nerve stimulation for faecal incontinence. Br J Surg 2008;95:1037–43.
136. El-Gazzaz G, Zutshi M, Salcedo L, et al. Sacral neuromodulation for the treatment of fecal incontinence and urinary incontinence in female patients: long-term follow-up. Int J Colorectal Dis 2009;24(12):1377–81.
137. Govaert B, Melenhorst J, Nieman FH, et al. Factors associated with percutaneous nerve evaluation and permanent sacral nerve modulation outcome in patients with fecal incontinence. Dis Colon Rectum 2009;52:1688–94.
138. Dudding TC, Pares D, Vaizey CJ, et al. Comparison of clinical outcome between open and percutaneous lead insertion for permanent sacral nerve neurostimulation for the treatment of fecal incontinence. Dis Colon Rectum 2009;52:463–8.
139. Altomare DF, Ratto C, Ganio E, et al. Long-term outcome of sacral nerve stimulation for fecal incontinence. Dis Colon Rectum 2009;52:11–7.
140. Michelsen HB, Thompson-Fawcett M, Lundby L, et al. Six years of experience with sacral nerve stimulation for fecal incontinence. Dis Colon Rectum 2010; 53:414–21.

141. Lombardi G, Del Popolo G, Cecconi F, et al. Clinical outcome of sacral neuromo-dulation in incomplete spinal cord-injured patients suffering from neurogenic bowel dysfunctions. Spinal Cord 2010;48:154–9.
142. Hollingshead JR, Dudding TC, Vaizey CJ. Sacral nerve stimulation for faecal in-continence: results from a single centre over a 10 year period. Colorectal Dis 2011;13:1030–4.
143. Santoro GA, Infantino A, Cancian L, et al. Sacral nerve stimulation for fecal in-continence related to external sphincter atrophy. Dis Colon Rectum 2012;55:797–805.
144. Duelund-Jakobsen J, van Wunnik B, Buntzen S, et al. Functional results and pa-tient satisfaction with sacral nerve stimulation for idiopathic faecal incontinence. Colorectal Dis 2012;14:753–9.
145. Devroede G, Giese C, Wexner SD, et al. SNS Study Group. Quality of life is markedly improved in patients with fecal incontinence after sacral nerve stimu-lation. Female Pelvic Med Reconstr Surg 2012;18:103–12.

Registries as Tools for Clinical Excellence and the Development of the Pelvic Floor Disorders Registry

CrossMark

Emily E. Weber LeBrun, MD, MS

KEYWORDS

- Pelvic floor disorders • Registry • Urogynecology • Pelvic reconstructive surgery
- Postmarket device surveillance • Surgical device innovation

KEY POINTS

- Historically, surgical device innovation has been less regulated than drug development, although the Food and Drug Administration (FDA) has recently initiated efforts to strengthen the national postmarket surveillance system through registry development.
- Device registries gather information about how patients respond after medical or surgical devices are used or implanted and can provide postmarket surveillance of new technologies and allow comparison with currently established treatments or devices.
- The Pelvic Floor Disorders Registry was developed in collaboration with the FDA, device manufacturers, and other stakeholders to serve as a platform for industry-sponsored postmarket device surveillance, investigator-initiated research, and quality and effectiveness benchmarking, all designed to improve the care of women with pelvic floor disorders.

INTRODUCTION

Innovation without analysis is perilous, and *convention* without analysis is stagnant.

The goals of healing are what drive our commitment to medical and surgical progress. However, advancements in pelvic reconstructive surgery are plagued by the same catch–22 that envelops all surgeons in turmoil. How do we expand therapeutic options without accepting risk? How do we predict outcomes without performing the experiment? How do we care for the individual who has entrusted her health to us with the confidence that we are providing her our very best? The answer lies in a universal commitment to perpetual, honest, and critical performance analysis.

The author has no financial or other disclosures.
Department of Obstetrics and Gynecology, University of Florida College of Medicine, 1600 Southwest Archer Road, PO Box 100294, Gainesville, FL 32610, USA
E-mail address: eweber@ufl.edu

Obstet Gynecol Clin N Am 43 (2016) 121–130
http://dx.doi.org/10.1016/j.ogc.2015.10.006
0889-8545/16/$ – see front matter © 2016 Elsevier Inc. All rights reserved.

obgyn.theclinics.com

HISTORY OF SURGICAL INNOVATION

Randomized controlled trials (RCTs) have gained status and stronghold as the gold standard for evaluating the safety and efficacy of surgical interventions.[1] Yet, most surgical advancements have been accepted from nonrandomized trials and even single case reports.[1] The reason for this internal conflict is time. In modern history, the development of endoscopic surgery for the removal of the diseased gall bladder was first performed in 1985, using a surgeon-designed instrument. However, it was not until 2006 that the Cochrane Collaboration provided a meta-analysis of 38 RCTs with 2338 patients that allowed the investigators to confirm the benefits of laparoscopic over open cholecystectomy.[2] In those 20 years, laparoscopic cholecystectomy had already been accepted as the preferred surgical approach worldwide. When it comes to RCTs, time is not on our side. Patients and surgeons alike have become accustomed to the ever-changing landscape of treatment options, driven largely by in-the-moment device and technique modifications that stealthily creep into standard practice.

Unlike new medical treatments that have followed a formalized development process from bench to bedside, surgical innovation has largely been unregulated because of immeasurable factors, including operator, team, setting, learning curves, and variations in quality metrics.[3] In 1976, the US Congress passed an amendment designed to provide some type of premarket review for medical devices, now monitored by the Center for Devices and Radiologic Health at the Food and Drug Administration (FDA). Novel devices are submitted for premarket approval (PMA) similar to a new drug, whereas design updates (even those from new manufacturers) request a simpler premarket notification (also called 510[k]), which is basically an expedited review based on reports of "equivalence to legally marketed predicate devices."[4,5] The PMA and 510(k) reviews provide clearance for marketing and sales of new medical devices and specifically do *not* indicate FDA clinical approval, *per se*. These premarket submissions are required to provide performance testing to demonstrate any deviations from the predicate device and may include engineering, bench, design verification, and, if requested by the FDA, clinical trials.[5] Once a device has cleared the 510(k) process, it may serve as a predicate device for subsequent 510(k) submissions; however, problems with effectiveness and safety are not readily apparent because postmarket trials are rare.[6]

Although innovations in medical device technologies have translated into significant health advances, the standard review process for medical/surgical devices is less stringent, less expensive, and faster than for drugs.[7] The role of surgical innovation in pelvic floor disorders follows the trajectory of other subspecialties: improving patient outcomes, leading to innovation and, in turn, leading to uncertain risk, a risk that is squarely shouldered by trusting patients. So, how do we responsibly and proactively integrate daily, ever-changing surgical innovation into safe and effective surgical advancement? *The answer lies in the power of the collective.*

REGISTRIES: THE POWER OF POOLING DATA

The emergence of medical and surgical registries to bolster our understanding of treatment outcomes has been evolving over the past 20 years or more with notable success. Patient registries use observational study methods for collecting uniform data to evaluate specific outcomes from a population defined by a particular disease, condition, or exposure.[8] Patient registries can be used to learn about population behavior patterns, develop research hypotheses, collect tissue or blood samples, monitor outcomes, and study best practices. Although the purposes of patient registries can vary widely, their utility has been recently propelled by federal quality-improvement initiatives, especially those related to the desire for health care costs to reflect quality. Historically, claims data provided the only determinants of quality; however, these databases were limited by misclassifications, omissions of complication severity, and the inability to produce risk adjustment.[9] Ideally, prospective surgical registries are designed for long-term data collection enhanced by a known case denominator to capture opportunities for quality improvement.

Two examples of successful surgical registries that use different approaches are the Society of Thoracic Surgeons (STS) and the Vascular Quality Initiative. The STS is a national database created as an initiative for quality improvement and patient safety among cardiothoracic surgeons and encompasses 3 distinct areas of surgery: adult cardiac, general thoracic, and congenital heart surgery. Although the original focus was quality improvement, the database has become a powerful tool for research, producing more than 100 publications to date. In addition, the STS continues to expand in scope, now allowing surgeon-participants to voluntarily report their surgical performance to the public. One branch of the database contains approximately 90% of all adult cardiac surgery centers across the United States; the STS has also expanded worldwide. The breadth of the STS has allowed it to provide valuable practice guidelines based on careful risk-adjustment and collective quality indicators reflective of the entire clinical care team.[9]

The Vascular Quality Initiative (VQI) has taken a different approach, building a distributed network of regional quality groups that operate under a single patient safety organization and use a cloud-based data-entry platform. The 18 regional quality groups allow for geographic, anonymous pooling of data, with the purpose of encouraging participants to initiate quality-improvement projects relevant to their patient population. Innovation in medical/surgical devices is a key component in vascular health care; the VQI invites device and drug manufacturers to leverage regulatory requirements for premarket and postmarket approval and improve quality of care.[10]

A relatively new project by the American College of Surgeons (ACS) features the first Surgeon Specific Registry (SSR), encouraging tracking of individual surgeon outcomes. This registry is extremely valuable for the rural or solo practitioner or those practicing in highly specialized fields who may be operating without consistent collegial support. The SSR has successfully integrated Maintenance of Certification Part 4 and recently became designated as a Quality Clinical Data Registry, which allows surgeons to benefit from federal quality-reporting incentives through SSR participation. The ACS invites pelvic floor surgeons to join the SSR and receive benchmark and real-time online reports.

Device registries gather information about how patients respond after medical or surgical devices are used or implanted. Registries can provide postmarket surveillance of new technologies and allow comparison with currently established treatments or devices. Clinical trials typically lack the funding for the data collection required for this type of long-term device performance assessment.[11] Orthopedics provides a valuable example of how hip implant registries were instrumental in identifying higher failure rates of metal-on-metal implants, reported by surgeons in comparison with other implants. This finding, in 2010, prompted the recall of 93,000 hip implants in Australia and the United Kingdom.[12,13] The voluntary American Joint Replacement Registry is tracking knee and hip implant surgeries at 535 hospitals by 4064 surgeons in 50 states.[14]

Federal government efforts to support prospective data collection through registries are taking a stronger hold. The FDA has now formed 2 groups toward this end. The National Medical Device Postmarket Surveillance System Planning Board will work to strengthen the postmarket surveillance process in the United States in order to identify problems with devices more quickly. The Medical Device Registry Task Force will address the topic of registry development in 5 ways (**Box 1**).[15] Although the FDA does not currently have the authority to require registry development and participation, reimbursement and coverage incentives through the Centers for Medicare and Medicaid Services (CMS) can encourage registry contribution. The goal of strengthening postmarket surveillance for medical devices is to protect and promote the public health through safety and efficacy assessment; registries provide the broad patient capture, real-world generalizability, scalable and reusable infrastructure, near real-time analysis, and structured, standardized data.[16]

INCREASING PREVALENCE OF PELVIC FLOOR DISORDERS

Pelvic floor disorders are now considered a common problem, affecting nearly 25% of adult women in the United States, the prevalence increasing with age.[17] Large, population-based research has improved our understanding of the impact that pelvic floor disorders have on the community, identifying as many as 20% of women presenting for surgical treatment by 80 years of age and up to one-third of those women undergoing 2 or more surgical procedures.[17,18] The demand for surgical prolapse repairs is predicted to increase by 35% over the next 30 years, placing even greater importance on developing evidenced-based standards of care.[19]

SURGICAL TREATMENT OF PELVIC ORGAN PROLAPSE

Surgery for pelvic organ prolapse (POP) continues to evolve from traditional native-tissue vaginal repair and open sacral colpopexy to a variety of surgical approaches, techniques, materials, and devices. Laparoscopic prolapse repairs were traditionally performed by a small subset of uniquely skilled surgeons who performed uterosacral suspension, paravaginal repair, and sacral colpopexy, among others. The purchase of surgical robots by hospitals and surgical centers, and their ease of use, has increased

---

Box 1
Primary objectives for the National Medical Device Registry Task Force

1. Identify existing registries that may contribute to a national medical device postmarket surveillance system.

2. Leverage on-going registry efforts focused on quality improvement, reimbursement, patient-centered outcomes, and other related activities to best meet the needs of multiple stakeholders.

3. Identify priority medical device types for which the establishment of a longitudinal registry is of significant public health importance, such as a subset of class III or permanently implantable class II medical devices.

4. Identify and prioritize successful registry governance and data quality best practices that promote rigorous design, conduct, analysis, and transparency to meet needs of stakeholders, including the FDA.

5. Develop strategies for the use of registries to support PMA and clearance as well as postmarket indication extensions in labeling.

Adapted from Medical Device Epidemiology Network: National Medical Device Registry Task Force. Available at: http://mdepinet.org/how-we-work/registry-task-force/. Accessed October 21, 2015.

the performance of robotic sacral colpopexy, making this minimally invasive option more accessible to surgeons with a spectrum of experience.[20] Now that laparoscopic surgery and robotic assistance is standard, surgeons have many different methods and techniques to offer when counseling patients about surgery for POP (**Table 1**). Interestingly, we have little data about how, and to what extent, surgeons present these options to their patients.

In a response to postoperative prolapse recurrence, combined with the typical innovation found in surgery, some of the new materials and devices integrated into pelvic reconstruction were borrowed from other disciplines without supporting evidence for these applications. The use of synthetic or biologic mesh augmentation for both vaginal and abdominal prolapse repairs was adopted from general surgery based on ventral hernia repair. The products were developed and incorporated into standard practice quite rapidly, as they provided the promise of improved durability packaged with a delivery system accessible to many pelvic surgeons. These products were cleared for sales by the FDA 510(k) process, with varying levels of clinical safety and efficacy data. So successful was the marketing for these techniques and materials that from 2005 to 2010, almost one-third of all prolapse repairs were augmented with mesh, and 75% of those were placed via a transvaginal approach.[21]

Although transvaginal mesh and sacral colpopexy may be perceived by some as exceptional one-size-fits-all procedures, many female pelvic medicine and reconstructive surgery (FPMRS) specialists continue to incorporate tailored approaches in their surgical practice, taking into account the individual patient's symptom profile, tissue quality, and treatment goals.

THE COLLAPSE OF THE TRANSVAGINAL MESH AND BUILDING OF NEW BRIDGES

Transvaginal mesh augmentation for POP surgery enjoyed a strong market presence in the United States until a spike in adverse events reported to the Manufacturer and

Table 1
The many surgical approaches, techniques, and device types available for repairing POP

		Route	
Segment	Surgical Approach	Transvaginal	Abdominal[a]
Anterior	Native tissue	Anterior colporrhaphy Paravaginal repair	Paravaginal repair
	Mesh augmented[a]	Free graft[a] Mesh kit[a]	Sacrocolpopexy[a]
Posterior	Native tissue	Posterior colporrhaphy	not applicable
	Mesh augmented[a]	Free graft[a] Mesh kit[a]	Sacrocolpopexy[a]
Apical	Native tissue	Vaginal vault suspension: • Uterosacral • Sacrospinous • Iliococcygeus	Abdominal vaginal vault suspension: • Uterosacral
	Mesh augmented[a]	Free graft[a] Mesh kit[a]	Sacrocolpopexy[a]
Obliterative (all compartments)	Native tissue	Colpocleisis	not applicable

[a] At least 6 different companies manufactured one or more device for use in pelvic reconstructive surgery.
Courtesy of M. Barber, MD, MHS, Cleveland, OH.

User Facility Device Experience (MAUDE) database prompted an investigation by the FDA. More than 1000 reports from 9 surgical mesh manufacturers were documented in the MAUDE database by 2005. The top 5 reported adverse events were mesh erosion (35.1%), pain (31.4%), infection (16.8%), bleeding (8.2%), and dyspareunia (7.2%). These reports prompted an ever-escalating cascade of responses from the FDA and private medical organizations, culminating in a dramatic change in surgical practice (**Box 2**).

In the year following the FDA safety communication, transvaginal mesh products sales experienced a decline of 70% and hundreds of lawsuits were filed nationwide. Although some surgeons continued to use the products, confident in their own outcomes, the public became increasingly aware of the problems associated with mesh, and subsequent incorporation of this information into the surgical consent process became quite challenging. Excellent and prompt leadership from several private medical organizations provided much needed recommendations and guidance to surgeons and patients alike. In addition, an unprecedented partnership developed between multiple private and federal stakeholders, hoping to better understand the role of mesh augmentation for POP repair.

Instead of removing the transvaginal mesh products from the market and, thus, eliminating a tool for POP surgery, in early 2012, the FDA ordered the urogynecologic surgical mesh manufacturers to enter their products into postmarket surveillance studies (called the 522 order). The FDA further recommended that these studies be performed within a prospective registry design and that they use native tissue prolapse repairs as a control group for comparison. The American Urogynecologic Society (AUGS), partnering with the FDA and device manufacturers, offered to design and host a registry that would serve the 522 order requirements and allow practicing surgeons to track their outcomes and report complications.[25] The project of creating the Pelvic Floor Disorders Registry (PFDR) rapidly became a tremendously complex, integrated work of patience, diligence, and trust between heretofore unlikely partners.

BUILDING A UNIVERSAL PELVIC FLOOR DISORDERS REGISTRY

Once the goals of the PFDR were established (**Box 3**), work on conceptualizing the registry, selecting data elements, and defining adverse events was undertaken by an AUGS task force that would later be divided into the registry's steering committee and scientific committee. In order to meet the primary objectives, the registry was soon divided into sections that would reflect the anticipated participation. The industry-sponsored (PFDR-I) database contains the robust requirements of the FDA 522 order and is flexible enough to accommodate the variety of data elements required by each industry partner for the multiple study protocols. Voluntary, physician-initiated participation (outside of the 522 order) evolved into 2 groups, separated mainly by research and quality goals. Surgeons interested in quality and research enroll in the PFDR - Research Registry, which contains most of the same data elements built for the PFDR-IS and engages patients through an informed-consent process, with the aim of contributing subjective, patient-reported outcomes over time. Surgeons committed primarily to quality improvement can access the PFDR–Quality Improvement Registry, in which they will be able to collect important quality indicators and benefit from collective benchmarking reports provided to all participants.

Some of the most notable challenges in creating the PFDR were related to the many stakeholders involved including device manufacturers, various government regulatory and research agencies, and surgeons and their associated professional

Box 2
Important dates in the evolution of the Pelvic Floor Disorders Registry

- 1996: Protegen by BSC (Marlborough, MA) was introduced as the first sling kit.

- 1998: Tension-free vaginal tape by Ethicon (Somerville, NJ) was introduced.

- 2001: IVS Tunneler by United States Surgical (now Covidien, Dublin, Ireland) was introduced as the first POP kit.

- 2004: Perigee by AMS (Marlborough, MA) was introduced in the United States, and the first study was performed; the first RCT was performed in 2008.

- 2005: Prolift by Ethicon was introduced in the United States, and the first study was done in 2006; the first RCT was performed in 2009.

- 2008: Elevate by AMS and Uphold by BSC were introduced in the United States; the first studies were done in 2012.

- 2005 to 2007: Increased adverse event signals from the MAUDE database triggered an FDA review of the data.

- 2008: FDA issued a public health notice regarding adverse events associated with surgical mesh when used for POP and SUI.

- 2008 to 2010: FDA performed a second review of the MAUDE database.

- July 2011: FDA released a safety communication indicating that complications from transvaginal mesh were not rare and efficacy over nonmesh repair was not clear.[23]

- September 2011: The FDA convened a meeting of the Obstetrics-Gynecology Devices Panel of the Medical Devices Advisory Committee to discuss the safety and efficacy of transvaginal placement of mesh for POP and SUI.

- December 2011: The Committee Opinion on Vaginal Placement of Synthetic Mesh for POP was published.[24] Recommendations were published by the AUGS and ACOG that strongly supported the development of a registry for postmarket surveillance.

- January 2012: The FDA ordered manufacturers of transvaginal mesh products for POP to conduct postmarket surveillance under Section 522 of the Federal Food, Drug, and Cosmetic Act (522 order) using a prospective registry design.

- March 2012: The AUGS agreed to collaborate with industry, the FDA, and other professional organizations (FDA, NICHD, ACOG, WHRA, PFDN Advisory Board, SUFU, AUA) to host a registry designed to meet both the 522 requirements and serve practicing surgeons.

- 2012 to 2015: Four device manufacturers (Acell, AMS, BSC, and Coloplast) partnered with the AUGS to develop the Pelvic Floor Disorders Registry.

- 2013: The FDA edited their 2011 safety communication with recommendations for surgeons and patients planning on a mesh-augmented prolapse repair.

Abbreviations: ACOG, American College of Obstetricians and Gynecologists; AMS, American Medical Systems; AUA, American Urologic Association; AUGS, American Urogynecologic Society; BSC, Boston Scientific; IVS, intra-vaginal sling; NICHD, Eunice Kennedy Shriver National Institute of Child Health and Human Development; PFDN, Pelvic Floor Disorders Network; SUFU, Society of Urodynamics, Female Pelvic Medicine, and Urogenital Reconstruction; SUI, stress urinary incontinence; WHRA, Women's Health Registry Alliance.
  Data from Refs.[22–24]

organizations.[25] The various industry partners were involved in designing multiple 522-ordered studies and shared concerns about project privacy, which initially interfered with collaboration but was eventually overcome by the sheer significance of the task. Predicting which outcome data will remain relevant in the future is always a challenge in prospective trials, as is anticipating the ever-changing data-collection

---

Box 3
Primary objectives for the PFDR

1. Evaluate the effectiveness, quality of life, and safety associated with surgical options (transvaginal/transabdominal native tissue repair, transvaginal mesh repair, and sacrocolpopexy) for POP

2. Assess the effectiveness and quality of life associated with nonsurgical management (pessary) for POP

3. Provide a framework for clinical studies to be conducted within the registry, including industry-sponsored studies required to fulfill the FDA's request for postmarketing surveillance for transvaginal mesh for POP

4. Allow providers to track surgical volume, patient characteristics, objective and subjective outcomes, patient-reported outcomes, adverse events (including rare patient events), and quality measures (CMS, PQRS, and maintenance of certification requirements)

5. Interface with the American Congress of Obstetricians and Gynecologists Women's Health Registry Alliance

---

platforms, especially given the goal for long-term patient-reported outcomes. Because of industry involvement, there were unique financial considerations and the need for efficient coordination of multiple protocols. The PFDR continues to work on integrating national quality measures; although it hopes to provide maintenance of certification for the FPMRS subspecialty, the goal is that surgeons with and without FPMRS board certification recognize the value in this collective resource.

The PFDR is now an active, online, multicentered, national prospective cohort study of patients undergoing treatment of POP that is designed to collect both provider- and patient-reported outcomes through broad participation from specialists and generalists performing surgery for prolapse.[26] As of January 2016, 236 sites and 646 surgeons have enrolled over 1500 patients into the PFDR. Although 522 industry-sponsored protocols account for most of that activity, a small group of surgeon volunteers (called Pioneer Sites) have received training and are actively enrolling patients. These Pioneer Sites will provide invaluable feedback regarding the site and patient enrollment process, which will improve the support provided by AUGS for future PFDR contributors. In just a short time, the PFDR has accumulated much prospective data from multiple sources. The variation in surgical practice and the drive toward innovation makes the PFDR well positioned to provide much-needed outcomes data on current and future surgical procedures.

SUMMARY

The integration of surgical and device registries into clinical research has begun a momentum toward a new era of surgical innovation, one in which every patient can contribute to global knowledge. Surgical registries harness the power of uniform data collection from varied sources to assess real-world clinical outcomes, treatment efficacy, and patient safety. These findings will enlighten the direction of surgical innovation and guide clinical and policy decision making.

There are significant barriers to registry development, most notably the costly and complex nature of registry design. The variability of electronic medical record (EMR) systems and concerns about privacy challenge the efforts to supplant parallel, duplicate data entry with automated EMR data extraction. To date, much of the registry development has been accomplished by the volunteer efforts of clinicians committed to a cause within their field. This effort has resulted in an assemblage of registries with varying missions, scope, designs, and success.

The ongoing goal of clinical excellence requires thorough, persistent, and honest self-assessment and transparency. The PFDR has opened a new chapter of outcomes assessment for patients and surgeons participating in pelvic reconstruction. Regardless of training, background, position, or caseload, any and all pelvic surgeons may participate in the PFDR, facilitated by a team of staff and volunteers aimed at providing access to quality-improvement strategies. Whether through a national or a local data repository, the gift of the human experience lies in the power to use information provided by a single patient to be analyzed in aggregate and then translated back to optimize the treatment of subsequent patients. Let the knowledge gained from mothers and sisters improve the care for their friends and daughters.

REFERENCES

1. Ergina PL, Cook JA, Blazeby JM, et al. Challenges in evaluating surgical innovation. Lancet 2009;374(9695):1097–104.
2. Kockerling F. The need for registries in the early scientific evaluation of surgical innovations. Front Surg 2014;1:12.
3. McCulloch P, Altman DG, Campbell WB, et al. No surgical innovation without evaluation: the IDEAL recommendations. Lancet 2009;374(9695):1105–12.
4. US Department of Health and Human Services, Food and Drug Administration. Device Approvals, Denials and Clearances. Available at: http://www.fda.gov/MedicalDevices/ProductsandMedicalProcedures/DeviceApprovalsandClearances/. Accessed September 2015.
5. US Department of Health and Human Services, Food and Drug Administration. The 510(k) Program: Evaluating Substantial Equivalence in Premarket Notifications [510(k)]. Available at: http://www.fda.gov/downloads/MedicalDevices/.../UCM284443.pdf. Accessed September 2015.
6. Hines JZ, Lurie P, Yu E, et al. Left to their own devices: breakdowns in United States medical device premarket review. PLoS Med 2010;7(7):e1000280.
7. Office GA. Medical devices: FDA should take steps to ensure that high-risk device types are approved through the most stringent premarket review process. Washington, DC: Government Printing Office; 2009. No. GAO-09-190.
8. Workman T. Engaging Patients in Information Sharing and Data Collection: The Role of Patient-Powered Registries and Research Networks. Rockville (MD): Agency for Healthcare Research and Quality (US); 2013 Sept. Available from: http://www.ncbi.nlm.nih.gov/sites/books/NBK164520/. Accessed September 2015.
9. Erekson EA, Iglesia CB. Improving patient outcomes in gynecology: the role of large data registries and big data analytics. J Minim Invasive Gynecol 2015; 22(7):1124–9.
10. Vascular Quality Initiative: Medical Device Evaluation Projects. Society for Vascular Surgery, Chicago, IL. Available at: http://www.vascularqualityinitiative.org/overview-benefits/medical-device-evaluation-projects/. Accessed September 2015.
11. Lee J. Groups press FDA to encourage medical-device registries. Modern Healthcare, September 3, 2014. Available at: http://www.modernhealthcare.com/article/20140903/NEWS/309039954. Accessed September 2015.
12. Australian Orthopaedic Association National Joint Replacement Registry. Annual Report 2010. Hip and Knee Arthroplasty, September 1999 to December 2009.

Available at: https://aoanjrr.dmac.adelaide.edu.au/documents/10180/42844/Annual%20Report%202010?version=1.1&t=1349406187793. Accessed September 2015.

13. National Joint Registry for England and Wales. 8th Annual Report 2010. Available at: http://www.njrcentre.org.uk/NjrCentre/Portals/0/Documents/NJR%208th%20Annual%20Report%202011.pdf. Accessed September 2015.

14. American Joint Replacement Registry: Improving Orthopaedic Care Through Data. Annual Report 2014. Available at: http://www.ajrr.net/images/annual_reports/AJRR_2014_Annual_Report_final.pdf. Accessed September 2015.

15. Medical Device Epidemiology Network. National Medical Device Registry Task Force. Available at: http://mdepinet.org/how-we-work/registry-task-force/. Accessed September 2015.

16. Strengthening our National System for Medical Device Postmarket Surveillance: Update and Next Steps. April 2013. Center for Devices and Radiological Health, US Food and Drug Administration. http://www.fda.gov/downloads/MedicalDevices/Safety/CDRHPostmarketSurveillance/UCM348845.pdf.

17. Nygaard I, Barber MD, Burgio KL, et al. Prevalence of symptomatic pelvic floor disorders in US women. JAMA 2008;300(11):1311–6.

18. Wu JM, Kawasaki A, Hundley AF, et al. Predicting the number of women who will undergo incontinence and prolapse surgery, 2010 to 2050. Am J Obstet Gynecol 2011;205(3):230.e1–5.

19. Vincent GK, Velkoff VA. The next four decades, the older population in the United States: 2010 to 2050. Washington DC: U.S. Census Bureau; May 2010. Available at: https://www.census.gov/prod/2010pubs/p25-1138.pdf. Accessed September 2015.

20. Brazell HD, O'Sullivan DM, Lasala CA. Trends in sacral colpopexy for the management of apical prolapse. Conn Med 2014;78(3):153–7.

21. Jonsson Funk M, Edenfield AL, Pate V, et al. Trends in use of surgical mesh for pelvic organ prolapse. Am J Obstet Gynecol 2013;208(1):79.e1–7.

22. Anderson-Smits C. Developing of the Pelvic Floor Disorders Registry (PFDR). US Food and Drug Administration. Available at: http://www.fda.gov/downloads/MedicalDevices/NewsEvents/WorkshopsConferences/UCM360236.pdf. Accessed September 2015.

23. Food and Drug Administration. Update on Serious Complications Associated with Transvaginal Placement of Surgical Mesh for Pelvic Organ Prolapse: FDA Safety Communication. July 13, 2011; US Food and Drug Administration. Available at: http://www.fda.gov/medicaldevices/safety/alertsandnotices/ucm262435.htm. Accessed September 2015.

24. American College of Obstetricians and Gynecologists. Vaginal placement of synthetic mesh for pelvic organ prolapse. Committee Opinion No. 513. Obstet Gynecol 2011;118(6):1459–64.

25. Bradley C, Visco AG, Weber LeBrun EE. The Pelvic Floor Disorders Registry (PFDR): Purpose and Development. Female Pelvic Med Reconstr Surg 2015. [Epub ahead of print].

26. Weber LeBrun EE, Adam RA, Barber MD, et al. The Pelvic Floor Disorders Registry (PFDR): study design and outcome measures. Female Pelvic Med Reconstr Surg. (ahead of print).

Informed Consent for Reconstructive Pelvic Surgery

Pakeeza Alam, MD[a],*, Cheryl B. Iglesia, MD[b,c]

KEYWORDS

- Informed consent - Urogynecology - Vaginal mesh - Female reconstructive surgery

KEY POINTS

- Informed consent is the process in which a patient makes a decision about a surgical procedure or medical intervention after adequate information about the procedure is relayed by his or her physician and understood by the patient.
- In the current medical legal environment, it is important to be well versed in obtaining valid informed consent for routine cases and for more complex procedures. This is critical for reconstructive pelvic surgeries particularly with the advent of vaginal mesh complications.
- In this article, we review the principles of informed consent, the pros and cons of different approaches in reconstructive pelvic surgery, and the current legal issues surrounding mesh use for vaginal surgery, and incorporate this information when consenting patients pelvic floor surgery.

The legal principle of informed consent before surgery was highlighted in a landmark case in the early 1900s in *Schloendorff v Society of New York Hospital*, in which a surgeon performed a hysterectomy without patient informed consent because of a concern for malignancy. Justice Benjamin Cardozo famously stated: "Every human being of adult years and sound mind has a right to determine what shall be done with his own body; and a surgeon who performs an operation without his patient's consent commits assault for which he is liable in damages."[1]

Although *Schloendorff v Society of New York Hospital* exemplifies an extreme case, the principles derived from this case are still applicable today. Informed consent is the

Disclosure: No disclosures.
[a] Female Pelvic Medicine and Reconstructive Surgery, MedStar Washington Hospital Center, Georgetown University, Washington, DC, USA; [b] Section of Female Pelvic Medicine and Reconstructive Surgery, Department of Obstetrics and Gynecology, National Center for Advanced Pelvic Surgery, Georgetown University School of Medicine, Washington, DC, USA; [c] Section of Female Pelvic Medicine and Reconstructive Surgery, Department of Urology, National Center for Advanced Pelvic Surgery, Georgetown University School of Medicine, Washington, DC, USA
* Corresponding author. 106 Irving Street, N.W. Physicians Office Building North Tower, Suite POB 405 South Washington, DC 20010-2975.
E-mail address: Pakeeza.a.alam@medstar.net

Obstet Gynecol Clin N Am 43 (2016) 131–139
http://dx.doi.org/10.1016/j.ogc.2015.10.010
0889-8545/16/$ – see front matter © 2016 Elsevier Inc. All rights reserved.

process in which a patient makes a decision about a surgical procedure or medical intervention after adequate information about the procedure is relayed by the physician and understood by the patient. Informed consent highlights the process of shared decision-making in the patient-provider relationship. In the current medical legal environment, it is important to be well versed in obtaining valid informed consent for routine cases and for more complex procedures.

Most reconstructive pelvic surgeries are elective, nonemergent, and aimed at improving quality of life, but still carry inherent material risks. Patients should have a good understanding of these risks and make a balanced decision between accepting the risks of surgery with the prospect of improvement in quality of life. The current controversy over the use of mesh in pelvic floor surgery poignantly exemplifies the importance of obtaining proper informed consent and is a topic that can be difficult to broach with patients. In this review, we aim to address fundamentals of obtaining general surgical consent and, specifically in the context of pelvic reconstructive surgery, choosing which type of reconstructive surgery is most appropriate for which patient, deciding when mesh use may be appropriate, discussing alternative treatments, and documenting the consent process.

OBJECTIVES

1. To list principles of informed consent
2. To acknowledge current legal issues associated with mesh use and discussion points related to informed consent.

INFORMED CONSENT

In 2009, the Committee of Ethics of the American College of Obstetricians and Gynecologists articulated 8 fundamental concepts about informed consent that should be applied to any surgery, including pelvic floor reconstructive surgery, summarized as follows[2]:

- "Obtaining informed consent for medical treatment, for participation in medical research, and for participation in teaching exercises involving students and residents is an ethical requirement that is partially reflected in legal doctrines and requirements."
- "Seeking informed consent expresses respect for the patient as a person."
- "Informed consent not only ensures the protection of the patient against unwanted medical treatment, but it also makes possible the patient's active involvement in her medical planning and care."
- "Communication is necessary if informed consent is to be realized, and physicians can and should help to find ways to facilitate communication not only in individual relations with patients but also in the structured context of medical care institutions."
- "Informed consent should be looked on as a process rather than a signature on a form."
- "Physicians should make every effort to incorporate a commitment to informed consent within a commitment to provide medical benefit to patients."
- "When informed consent by the patient is impossible, a surrogate decision maker should be identified to represent the patient's wishes or best interests."
- "Physicians should acquaint themselves with federal and state requirements for informed consent. Physicians also should be aware of the policies within their own practices because these may vary from institution to institution."

These concepts can be applied to the 5 main steps of obtaining a valid consent:

A. Determine whether the patient has capacity to make an informed decision
B. Determine whether the patient is giving consent of his or her own free will
C. Disclosing the risks, benefits, and alternatives to a treatment
D. Determine the patient's comprehension of the consent discussion
E. Making a decision on how to proceed with treatment

Determining Capacity

A patient has capacity when she understands the significance of her situation and possible treatments, can apply this information rationally to make a decision, and can express choice. If it seems that the patient may not have capacity to make decisions about surgery, the physician is responsible for seeking out an appropriate surrogate. The following are some examples of when a provider should increase vigilance about assessing a patient's mental capacity: when the patient seems to have an abrupt change in mental status; when she is disagreeing with the recommended treatment; if she hastily consents to a particularly invasive surgery without significant consideration of risks and benefits; and if the patient has a known psychological or neurologic condition that could impair her judgment.[3,4]

Freely Consenting

It is often helpful for patients to remember the consent discussion when other family members are present, such as a spouse or other family member or acquaintance; however, the physician should determine and ensure that the patient is freely consenting without coercion or persuasion from others.

Disclosing Information

When providing patients with information about pelvic reconstructive surgery, the first step is to review the indication for the surgery or procedure. Indications and diagnoses are reviewed once a full evaluation of the patient has been performed, including detailed history and physical examination, a description of extent of anatomic abnormalities based on pelvic examination and preoperative testing, including evaluation for occult urinary incontinence. When simplified, the main indication for surgical repair of pelvic organ prolapse (POP) relates to the extent of bother to the patient or whether there is bladder or bowel dysfunction, sexual dysfunction, impact on body image, or negative impact on ability to engage in physical and social activities. Patients also should be offered pessary or expectant management (watchful waiting) because prolapse is a non–life-threatening condition, but may potentially progress.

The next step is to review the pros and cons of different approaches to POP surgery. To simplify this for patients, it may be reasonable to break it down to either native tissue repair or graft augmented repairs. Native tissue repair encompasses anterior repair (AR) and posterior repair, sacrospinous ligament fixation (SSLF), uterosacral ligament suspension (USLS), McCall culdoplasty, and the obliterative procedures colpocleisis and LeFort colpocleisis. When describing graft augmentation, the surgeon must distinguish vaginal from abdominal grafts. Graft material can be classified into synthetic, mesh, xenografts, or allografts. For pelvic reconstructive procedures, synthetic mesh grafts are the most commonly used and most studied. It is crucial to make the distinction between different types of mesh used in pelvic floor surgery. Patients will often associate the complications of vaginal mesh with that of mesh used for slings and sacrocolpopexy. Transvaginal mesh may be used for anterior, posterior, and/or apical prolapse. Mesh used in the abdomen, on the other hand, is used for sacrocolpopexy or hysteropexy, and is used to treat primarily apical prolapse but may also simultaneously correct anterior, posterior, and paravaginal defects. Last, mesh used for slings is significantly smaller than mesh used in vaginal and abdominal surgery and has very low erosion rates.[5] The American Urogynecologic Society (AUGS) and the Society of Urodynamic, Female Pelvic Medicine, and Urogenital Reconstruction have issued a patient-oriented handout that addresses frequently asked questions relating to mesh used in sling procedures that is useful to provide to patients to help them better distinguish this mesh from that used in prolapse repair (http://www.augs.org/p/bl/et/blogaid=194).[6]

It is important to detail benefits and risks. When discussing the success rates of surgery for POP, it is often easier for patients to understand surgical outcomes or effectiveness. Most surgeons quote success rates from the literature, as they are unaware of their own success rates and most physicians cannot accurately self-assess their surgical ability. Furthermore, patients who have failed prolapse surgery (eg, prolapse recurrence noted) often do not return to the same surgeon. Some would argue that surgeon report cards would be one way to approach this and increase transparency in tracking surgical outcomes. This type of audit process is in place for cardiac surgeons through national registries of commonly performed procedures, such as coronary artery bypass surgery, and the data from these registries are available to the public.[7,8] Although the goal of report cards is to increase transparency and promote the practice of evidence-based medicine as well as to track surgeon-specific outcomes, there are several drawbacks. Surgeon report cards may lead physicians to practice defensive medicine, would require risk-adjusted mortality rates, and the training of new surgeons would be jeopardized. Participation in the new AUGS Pelvic Floor Disorders Registry may be one way that pelvic reconstructive surgeons could track their outcomes (http://www.pfdr.org/).

The next step is to discuss expectations for recovery and when to follow up. Start by distinguishing whether surgery will require an overnight stay or whether the patient can go home on the same day. With pelvic floor surgery, especially with apical/anterior wall correction and surgery for incontinence, patients often do not realize that they will need to have a Foley catheter and a void trial before discharge. It is important to discuss the chance of potentially going home with a Foley catheter if the voiding trial is not successful and that additional follow-up is needed for removal in the office.

For the surgery itself, discuss who the participants will be in the surgery in addition to the surgeon. If the surgery will be performed at a teaching institution, the physician should ensure the patient realizes that there may be students, residents, and fellows involved in the case so that they are not taken by surprise on the day of surgery.

Finally, it is necessary to explain one's experience with the surgery. If the surgeon has never performed a procedure or does very few cases per year, it may be appropriate to refer to a specialist who is adept in the surgery or have another surgeon present who can act as a preceptor. Higher-volume surgeons in general have better outcomes and fewer complications.[9,10] This concept holds true with pelvic floor surgery as well. In a retrospective cohort study examining the incidence of mesh removal or revision after synthetic mesh sling procedure for stress urinary incontinence, lower volume surgeons had a 37% increased likelihood of complications.[11] According to Sung and colleagues,[12] women undergoing urogynecological surgery by low-volume surgeons experienced mortality rates 2.75 times higher than for those who had surgery performed by high-volume surgeons.

Patient Understanding

When disclosing information pertaining to surgery, it is important to minimize the use of medical terminology. Certain concepts and surgeries in pelvic floor reconstruction are difficult to visualize and understand. Several resources are available online, such as the Boston Scientific Pelvic Floor Institute (http://www.bostonscientific.com/en-US/medical-specialties/female-pelvic-medicine/pelvic-floor-institute.html) programs that can assist with visual renditions.[13] To gauge a patient's comprehension, it may be helpful to ask her to verbalize her understanding of the surgical procedure, risks, benefits, and alternatives. Oftentimes, the consent process requires multiple visits. Interestingly, when examining patient recall about mesh use in midurethral sling placement, one study found that there was a significant decline in patient recall about the use of mesh for the surgery as well as the risk of erosion when they were surveyed 6 weeks after initial surgery.[14] This findings suggests the possible need to reiterate risks and complications to patients on more than one occasion before surgery.

Decision

Although the physician should provide all the aforementioned information, the ultimate decision to proceed with surgery rests with the patient. The physician can make a treatment recommendation of one surgery over the other, but cannot tell patients which surgery to choose. When providing recommendations, physicians must also guard against influencing patients toward one procedure over another that would potentially result in financial gain.[15]

SURGICAL APPROACH

Pelvic floor reconstructive surgery may be approached through a variety of different routes, including vaginally, abdominally, laparoscopically, and robotically; may be done with or without mesh; may be done with or without a concomitant anti-incontinence procedure; and may be obliterative in nature. Several factors must be considered when deciding on approach. The first factor is the patient's goal(s) for surgery. The next factor is medical history and comorbidities. If a patient has had several previous abdominal surgeries or is extremely obese (body mass index that is ≥ 40 kg/m^2), one must be cautious in offering a laparoscopic approach.[16] If a laparoscopic approach is attempted, the patient should be informed of the risk for bleeding, organ injury, especially if there are adhesions, and the need for an abdominal incision. Alternative surgery in the event this happens should be discussed with the patient, such as vaginal, open, or robotic approaches. For patients with endometrial cancer and morbid obesity, a robotic approach tends to have fewer postoperative complications (ie, wound dehiscence and infection) compared with laparotomy[17]; however, few comparative trials among open, laparoscopic, and robotic pelvic reconstructive surgeries exist. Special consideration regarding complications from mesh use are given to those with increased risk of poor wound healing and infection, including uncontrolled diabetes, immunosuppression (either from medications, such as chronic steroids, or conditions, such as human immunodeficiency virus), tobacco use, or connective tissue disorders (ie, Ehlers-Danlos syndrome).

Urodynamic studies can help determine whether a patient may benefit from a concomitant incontinence surgery, such as a sling or a Burch. Over the years, the midurethral sling has been the treatment of choice for the treatment of stress urinary incontinence given its less invasive nature and equivalent outcomes compared with autologous slings and retropubic urethropexy procedures.[18,19] The synthetic midurethral sling is the preferred method if the primary POP surgery is through a vaginal route; however, a Burch procedure may be considered if the patient will be undergoing a laparoscopic or abdominal repair. For patients with prolapse and no stress urinary incontinence symptoms, a risk calculator is available that will predict the woman's risk of developing de novo incontinence based on age, body mass index, parity, diabetes history, and symptoms (http://www.r-calc.com/ExistingFormulas.aspx?filter=CCQHS).[20]

Whether a patient is sexually active or not will also determine surgical approach. For patients who are not sexually active and who have no desire to become so in the future, obliterative procedures, such as a colpocleisis or colpectomy, have been found to be highly effective and are not as invasive as other pelvic floor surgeries.[21,22] This surgery is also a good option for patients who cannot be under general anesthesia for prolonged periods of time. Given their shorter operative times, obliterative surgeries also can be performed under regional anesthesia, such as a spinal and local anesthetic.

Finally, a patient's occupation and daily activities may make one surgical approach more optimal than another. For patients who are very active or who engage in heavy lifting for their occupation, a procedure that offers the highest cure rate, such as a sacrocolpopexy, may be the best option.

CONTROVERSY OF VAGINAL MESH

Vaginal mesh first appeared on the market in the late 1990s for anti-incontinence procedures. In the early 2000s, mesh implants for prolapse were developed with the idea that vaginal mesh would augment repairs to improve long-term effectiveness and durability of the repair. Vaginal synthetic mesh is predominantly used for ARs, but transvaginal mesh and mesh kits have evolved to target posterior as well as apical prolapse. Following a Food and Drug Administration (FDA) ObGyn devices panel meeting on vaginal mesh in September 2011, new orders (522 orders) were issued to manufacturers of vaginal mesh regarding increased postmarket surveillance of vaginal mesh kits for prolapse. National organizations, such as the American College of Obstetricians and Gynecologists (ACOG) and the AUGS, have come forward with position statements emphasizing the need for prospective postmarket surveillance studies on vaginal mesh and clinical trials for premarket requirement for transvaginal mesh use in prolapse repair.[23–25] AUGS insists that providers who use transvaginal mesh should be extensively trained in pelvic surgery, have a high volume of prolapse repairs, and be specifically trained in mesh and device handling. Furthermore, there must be comprehensive informed consent before use.[26] Several "522" or postmarket surveillance studies are currently being conducted investigating the long-term efficacy and safety for transvaginal mesh devices. In 2014, the FDA proposed to reclassify vaginal mesh used for POP surgery from a class II device to a class III device so that more rigorous premarketing prospective trials will be conducted for future transvaginal mesh products.[27]

The most common complications seen with mesh use include vaginal mesh exposure: pelvic pain, groin pain, and dyspareunia. Other complications include mesh contracture, scarring, and narrowing of the vaginal wall.[28,29] Current evidence shows improved anatomic outcomes when mesh is used in the anterior wall, but without improvement in quality of life. There are no high-quality studies that support the routine use of mesh graft in the posterior wall or for transvaginal apical support.[27]

When counseling patients before the use of mesh, the surgeon must review these risks but also emphasize that prospective studies are being conducted to better elucidate these risks. Until more prospective data are available, surgeons should be very selective when choosing candidates for transvaginal mesh placement, and this surgery may be reserved for patients who have recurrent prolapse, particularly in the anterior compartment.[30] As mentioned previously, vaginal mesh should be avoided in patients who do have other risks that would decrease wound healing and increase infection, such as immunosuppression and uncontrolled diabetes.

CURRENT LEGAL ENVIRONMENT

The FDA public heath notification and Update have spawned numerous lawsuits regarding mesh complications. Given the factual similarities between cases stemming from these complications, the lawsuits have resulted in multidistrict litigation[31] and the use of bellwether trials[32] to facilitate settlements against a manufacturer en masse. When plaintiff lawyers target manufacturers, there is incentive for a higher monetary settlement. However, in a recent review about the structure of these lawsuits, Kuhlmann-Capek and colleagues[33] explain why both manufacturers and surgeons may be targets. When naming a surgeon in a claim, the case is more likely to proceed in a local county or state court in which the plaintiff lawyer is more familiar. Additionally, in these civil suits when both manufacturer and surgeon are named as defendants, they will often be compelled to testify or otherwise adopt competing positions against each other. This scenario strengthens a plaintiff's case should the case proceed to a jury trial.

For plaintiff attorneys to claim medical malpractice, they must demonstrate that medical injury from mesh use occurred as a result of the physician's actions, either due to negligence or lack of informed consent. When negligence is claimed, the plaintiff attorney must prove that the physician used the mesh implant improperly and, therefore, strayed from the standard of care. If lack of informed consent is alleged, the plaintiff attorney must prove that had a reasonable person in the same circumstance as the patient been adequately consented, they would not have proceeded with the surgery.[34]

Manufacturers may transfer blame to surgeons in a claim of learned intermediary doctrine, in which manufacturers have provided physicians with all relevant information, including risks of complications and, therefore, have fulfilled their duty of care to the patient. It is then the duty of the "learned intermediary" to share this information with patients.[35]

Comprehensive, complete, and well-documented informed consent is critical in claims against the surgeon by plaintiff and by manufacturers. It is the physician's duty to become very familiar with mesh product manufacturer's labels and keep abreast with current studies with that particular product so as to provide adequate and accurate information when obtaining consent. It is equally critical to be aware of arguments made against surgeons in mesh litigation if they are named in a lawsuit.

SUMMARY

The informed consent process related to pelvic reconstructive surgery for prolapse includes a discussion of a patient's diagnoses, degree of bother, impact on physical and social activity, patient goals, surgeon experience, treatment options (both nonsurgical and surgical), and the option of expectant management. The process may need to incorporate visual aids, available prediction tools (risk calculators), and a discussion of limited outcome data for certain procedures. Patients should be made aware of ongoing clinical trials, and surgeons should consider enrollment in the AUGS Pelvic Floor Disorders Registry for native tissue repair, pessary management, and mesh-augmented surgeries.

REFERENCES

1. Schloendorff v Society of New York Hospital, 11 NY 125, 105 NE 92 (NY Ct App 1914).
2. ACOG Committee on Ethics. Informed consent. ACOG Committee Opinion No. 439. Obstet Gynecol 2009;114:401–8.
3. Bernat JL, Peterson LM. Patient-centered informed consent in surgical practice. Arch Surg 2006;141:86–92.
4. Tunzi M. Can patient decide? Evaluating patient capacity in practice. Am Fam Physician 2001;64(2):299–308.
5. Ford AA, Rogerson L, Cody JD, et al. Mid-urethral sling operations for stress urinary incontinence in women. Cochrane Database Syst Rev 2015;(7):CD006375.
6. Nager C, Tulikangas P, Miller D, et al. Frequently asked questions by patients: mid-urethral slings for stress urinary incontinence. AUGS/SUFU/MUS Task Force. 2014. Available at: http://www.augs.org/p/bl/et/blogaid=194. Accessed October 14, 2015.
7. Jha AK, Epstein AM. The predictive accuracy of the New York State coronary artery bypass surgery report-card system. Health Aff 2006;25(3):844–55.
8. Brown DL, Clarke S, Oakley J. Cardiac surgeon report cards, referral for cardiac surgery, and the ethical responsibilities of cardiologists. J Am Coll Cardiol 2012; 59:2378–82.
9. Birkmeyer JD, Siewers AE, Finlayson EVA, et al. Hospital volume and surgical mortality in United States. N Engl J Med 2002;346:1128–37.
10. Katz JN, Losina E, Barrett J, et al. Association between hospital and surgeon procedure volume and outcomes of total hip replacement in the United States Medicare population. J Bone Joint Surg Am 2001;83(11):1622–9.
11. Welk B, Al-Hothi H, Winick-Ng J. Removal or revision of vaginal mesh used for the treatment of stress urinary incontinence. JAMA Surg 2015;150(12):1167–75. Available at: http://archsurg.jamanetwork.com/article.aspx?articleid52432613. Accessed October 13, 2015.
12. Sung VW, Rogers ML, Myers DL, et al. Impact of hospital and surgeon volumes on outcomes following pelvic reconstructive surgery in the United States. Am J Obstet Gynecol 2006;195(6):1778–83.
13. Pelvic Floor Institute. Boston scientific and educare. 2014. Available at: http://www.bostonscientific.com/en-US/medical-specialties/female-pelvic-medicine/pelvic-floor-institute.html. Accessed October 14, 2015.
14. McFadden BL, Constantine ML, Hammil SL, et al. Patient recall 6 weeks after surgical consent for midurethral sling using mesh. Int Urogynecol J 2013;24:2099–104.
15. American College of Obstetricians and Gynecologists. Surgery and patient choice. ACOG Committee Opinion No. 395. Obstet Gynecol 2008;111:243–7.
16. The practical guide: identification, evaluation, and treatment of overweight and obesity in adults. US Department of Health and Human Services, Public Health Service, National Health Institutes, National Heart, Lung, and Blood Institute; 2000.
17. Bernardini MQ, Gien LT, Tipping H, et al. Surgical outcome of robotic surgery in morbidly obese patient with endometrial cancer compared to laparotomy. Int J Gynecol Cancer 2012;22(1):76–81.
18. Weber AM, Walters MD. Burch procedure compared with sling for stress urinary incontinence: a decision analysis. Obstet Gynecol 2000;96(6):867–73.
19. Bandarian M, Ghanbari Z, Asgari A. Comparison of transobdurator tape (TOT) vs Burch method in treatment of stress urinary incontinence. J Obstet Gynaecol 2011;31(6):518–20.

20. Risk of de novo postoperative stress urinary incontinence after surgery for pelvic organ prolapse. Publically published calculators – Cleveland Clinic. 2012. Available at: http://www.r-calc.com/ExistingFormulas.aspx?filter=CCQHS. Accessed October 14, 2015.
21. Zebede S, Smith AL, Plowright LN, et al. Obliterative LeFort colpocleisis in a large group of elderly women. Obstet Gynecol 2013;121(2 Pt 1):279–84.
22. Arunkalaivanan A, Ghosh A. Colpocleisis: a good option for the management of pelvic organ prolapse in selected elderly women. Int Urogynecol J Pelvic Floor Dysfunct 2006;17(3):261–71.
23. Society of Gynecologic Surgeons (SGS) executive committee statement regarding the FDA communication: surgical placement of mesh to repair pelvic organ prolapse imposes risks. Society of Gynecologic Surgeons; 2011. Available at: http://www.augs.org/p/cm/ld/fid=174. Accessed October 14, 2015.
24. NAFC position statement on the use of vaginal mesh in pelvic surgery. National Association for Continence; 2011. Available at: http://www.augs.org/p/cm/ld/fid=174. Accessed October 14, 2015.
25. American College of Obstetricians and Gynecologists. Vaginal placement of synthetic mesh for pelvic organ prolapse and urinary incontinence. ACOG Committee Opinion No. 513. Obstet Gynecol 2011;118(6):1459–64.
26. AUGS Position Statement on Restriction of Surgical Options of PFDs. 2013. Available at: http://www.augs.org/p/cm/ld/fid=174. Accessed October 14, 2015.
27. US Food and Drug Administration. Reclassification of surgical mesh for transvaginal pelvic organ prolapse repair and surgical instrumentation for urogynecologic surgical mesh procedures; designation of special controls for urogynecologic surgical mesh instrumentation. 2014. Available at: https://www.federalregister.gov/articles/2014/05/01/2014-09907/reclassification-of-surgical-mesh-for-transvaginal-pelvic-organ-prolapse-repair-and-surgical. Accessed October 14, 2015.
28. Maher C, Feiner B, Baessler K, et al. Surgical management of pelvic organ prolapse in women: a Cochrane review. Cochrane Database Syst Rev 2013;(4):CD004014.
29. Velemir L, Amblard J, Fatton B, et al. Transvaginal mesh repair of anterior and posterior vaginal wall prolapse: a clinical and ultrasonographic study. Ultrasound Obstet Gynecol 2010;35:474–80.
30. Murphy M. Clinical practice guidelines on vaginal graft use from the Society of Gynecologic Surgeons. Obstet Gynecol 2008;112(5):1123–30.
31. Multidistrict litigation, 28 U.S.C.S. § 1407. 2015.
32. Fallon EE, Grabill JT, Wynne RP. Bellwether trials in multidistrict litigation. Tulane Law Rev 2008;82:2323.
33. Kuhlmann-Capek MJ, Kilic GS, Shah AB, et al. Enmeshed in controversy: use of vaginal mesh in the current medicolegal environment. Female Pelvic Med Reconstr Surg 2015;21:241–3.
34. Ball SB. An introduction to medical malpractice in the United States. Clin Orthop Relat Res 2009;467(2):339–47.
35. Plant NK. The learned intermediary doctrine: some new medicine for an old ailment. Iowa Law Rev 1995–1996;81:1007.

Ultrasound Imaging of the Pelvic Floor

Daniel E. Stone, MD, Lieschen H. Quiroz, MD*

KEYWORDS

- Ultrasound • Vaginal ultrasound • Endoluminal ultrasound • Endoanal ultrasound

KEY POINTS

- Ultrasound is a detailed anatomic assessment of the muscles and surrounding organs of the pelvic floor.
- Anatomic variability and pathology, such as prolapse, fecal incontinence, urinary incontinence, vaginal wall cysts, synthetic implanted material, and pelvic pain, can be easily assessed with endoluminal vaginal ultrasound.
- Knowledge of pelvic floor anatomy is essential for effective ultrasound imaging techniques.

INTRODUCTION

The pelvic floor is a complex system, and adequate assessment of pelvic floor disorders is greatly supplemented by pelvic floor imaging. Rather than focusing on the clinical examination of pelvic floor surface structures, imaging modalities, such as sonography, allow for immediate, real-time confirmation of anatomic findings. Pelvic floor ultrasound offers a low cost, minimally invasive method of assessing pelvic floor anatomy and function. For example, clinical assessment of the anatomy of the levator ani by palpation requires significant skill and teaching.[1–3] Clinical diagnosis by imaging has been shown to be more reproducible than palpation and provides a more objective method of teaching.[3]

PELVIC FLOOR ANATOMY

The female pelvic floor and the levator ani complex are composed of muscle fibers and a fascial network, which spans the area underneath the pelvis. An intact, well-innervated pelvic floor is necessary to maintain pelvic organ support, facilitate

Disclosures: royalties from UpToDate (L.H. Quiroz).
Department of Obstetrics and Gynecology, University of Oklahoma Health Sciences Center, 920 Stanton L. Young, WP2430, Oklahoma City, OK 73104, USA
* Corresponding author.
E-mail address: Lieschen-Quiroz@ouhsc.edu

Obstet Gynecol Clin N Am 43 (2016) 141–153
http://dx.doi.org/10.1016/j.ogc.2015.10.007
0889-8545/16/$ – see front matter © 2016 Elsevier Inc. All rights reserved.

obgyn.theclinics.com

urination and defecation, and allow childbirth. The pelvic floor muscle hammock, or levator ani complex, is comprised of five distinguishable subdivisions, based on MRI studies (**Fig. 1**).[4,5] The pubovaginalis muscle arises from the posterior aspect of the pubic rami and inserts in the anterior vaginal wall at the level of the midurethra. The puborectalis muscle arises from the posterior aspect of the pubic ramus and runs posteriorly to form a sling around the rectum. During childbirth the puborectalis sustains the most stretch in vaginal delivery.[6] The puboperinealis muscle arises from the posterior aspect of the pubic rami and bilaterally inserts in the contralateral side of the perineal body. The puboanalis muscle arises from the posterior aspect of the pubic rami and inserts into the intersphincteric groove between the internal anal sphincter (IAS) and external anal sphincter (EAS). The iliococcygeus muscle arises from the arcus tendineus levator ani and runs medially to fuse at the midline in the iliococcygeal raphe. An intact pelvic floor muscle hammock functions to keep the urogenital hiatus closed by compressing the vagina, urethra, and rectum against the pubic bone during contraction.

The pelvic organs and levator ani muscle complex are encased by a dense network of endopelvic fascia. This network aids in pelvic organ support and keeps the pelvic organs in proper orientation during daily activities. Innervation of the pelvic floor is provided through the pudendal nerve and sacral nerve plexus arising from L4-S5. The pudendal nerve primarily innervates the anal and urethral sphincter, thus controlling the continence mechanisms. The levator ani nerve innervates the major musculature that supports the pelvic floor. The sacral nerve plexus is a distal component of the lumbosacral plexus and innervates the levator ani complex.

Knowledge of pelvic floor anatomy is essential for effective ultrasound imaging techniques. Advancing ultrasound technologies have improved the ability to detect pelvic floor defects and gain insight into the pathophysiology of pelvic floor disorders.

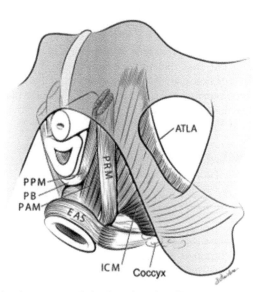

Fig. 1. Musculoskeletal anatomy of the female pelvic floor. ATLA, arcus tendineus levator ani; EAS, external anal sphincter; ICM, iliococcygeus muscle; PAM, puboanalis muscle; PB, perineal body; PPM, puboperinealis muscle; PRM, puborectalis muscle. (*From* Kearney R, Sawhney R, DeLancey JO. Levator ani muscle anatomy evaluated by origin-insertion pairs. Obstet Gynecol 2004;104:172; with permission.)

ULTRASOUND TECHNIQUE
Transperineal Ultrasound

Requirements for two-dimensional (2D) perineal ultrasound include a B-mode-capable 2D ultrasound system, and a 3.5- to 6-MHz transducer.[7] To perform the examination, the patient is placed in dorsal lithotomy position after the patient voids. The probe may be covered with a nonpowdered glove or probe cover. Ultrasound gel is applied to the probe and the probe is placed firmly on the perineum. Once a midsagittal view is obtained, the following structures should be identified from ventral to dorsal: symphysis pubis, urethra and bladder neck, vaginal canal, uterus and cervix, anorectal canal, and the central portion of the puborectalis muscle. Parting the labia may improve image quality. By rotating the probe 90°, one can obtain a coronal view and by placing a dorsal inclination on the probe, the anal canal and sphincter complex are seen and assessed. Once adequate images are obtained, the probe is removed from the perineum and cleaned.

2D images can be integrated into three-dimensional (3D) volume data either by a free-hand acquisition of images or using a probe equipped with a motor to allow for motorized automatic acquisition of images. To perform the examination the patient is in the same position as described for 2D ultrasound. Ultrasound gel is applied to the 3D-capable probe and placed firmly on the perineum in a midsagittal orientation. The probe is then held in place while the images are obtained. Postprocessing of the images then occurs and is evaluated with the appropriate software.[8] Four-dimensional imaging refers to the real-time acquisition of data to produce and save cineloops of the images obtained. To perform four-dimensional imaging, one must record images during a prompted maneuver, such as a squeeze or a Valsalva.

Endoluminal Ultrasound

Although a fair amount of information is obtained with an abdominal 2D probe when placed on the perineum (in the technique detailed previously), additional information is obtained by endoluminal ultrasound (endovaginal and endoanal ultrasound) with such equipment as the BK Medical Pro Focus Ultra View and Flex Focus (Peabody, MA). These systems provide high performance with efficiency and speed, high resolution, and a sensitive color Doppler with great spatial resolution and sensitivity.

Endovaginal ultrasound is performed with the patient in the dorsal lithotomy position, with the patient having a comfortable amount of urine in the bladder. Multiple types of probes are used including an electronic biplane 5- to 12-MHz probe, a high multifrequency 9- to 16-MHz probe, a 360° rotational mechanical probe, or with a radial electronic probe,[9,10] such as the one by BK Medical. To perform the examination, the transducer is inserted into the vagina in a neutral position, avoiding excessive pressure on the surrounding structures. The biplane electronic probe provides 2D imaging of the anterior and posterior compartments. Typically it is performed at rest, on Valsalva, and during pelvic floor muscle contraction. 3D images are obtained by connecting this transducer to an external 180° rotational mover. Other methods of obtaining 3D images are using a radial electronic probe or a rotational mechanical probe to obtain a 3D 360° view image of the pelvic floor. The 3D volume can be used on the scanner, but the better functionality is to use the free software, which can be installed in any personal computer. This allows for the volume to be exported to a CD, DVD, USB, or external drive and be viewed and analyzed at any time. The available functions of the software allow for manipulation of the 3D cube in the x, y, or z planes, and obtaining linear, angle, area, and volume measurements.

Endoanal Ultrasound

Endoanal ultrasound is the gold standard for evaluating anal sphincter pathology.[11] It is performed with the patient either in dorsal lithotomy, left lateral, or prone position. It can be performed either with a high multifrequency 360° rotational probe or a radial electronic probe. Irrespective of patient positioning, the transducer should be positioned so that the anterior aspect of the anal canal is superior on the screen at the 12-o'clock position. The distal end of the probe should be at the level of the puborectalis muscle or 6 cm into the anal canal. The mechanical rotational probe, once activated, automatically obtains 3D images.[9] 3D image acquisition with the radial electronic probe involves manual withdrawal.[12]

CLINICAL UTILITY

This discussion is focused on the clinical use of ultrasound imaging of the pelvic floor mostly to endoluminal ultrasound. Although pelvic floor imaging can be initiated with a transperineal ultrasound, having the advantage of dynamic imaging with minimal tissue distortion, the resulting images have a lower resolution.

Anterior Compartment

The anterior compartment of the pelvis is often assessed with transperineal and endovaginal ultrasound. Because there is an inherent displacement of tissue with endovaginal ultrasound, transperineal ultrasound is preferred for visualization of bladder neck descent, urethral hypermobility, cystocele, and cystourethrocele.[13] 3D endovaginal ultrasound is used to provide a detailed anatomic depiction of anterior compartment structures including the trigone, compressor urethra, and the urogenital sphincter.[14] 3D endovaginal ultrasound also allows the examiner to accurately measure the components of the urethral complex including urethral width, length, and volume.[9,14] **Fig. 2** Shows an example of normal urethral anatomy, including the striated urogenital

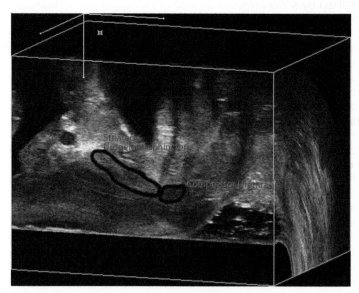

Fig. 2. Example of normal urethral anatomy, including the striated urogenital sphincter and compressor urethra as seen in this 3D endovaginal ultrasound.

sphincter and compressor urethra. It is an excellent tool for visualizing anterior vaginal cysts and masses including Skene gland cysts, urethral diverticula, and Gartner duct cysts.[15]

The female urethra is a complex organ that plays a central role in urinary incontinence. Normal anatomy, innervation, position, and proper relation to the surrounding pelvic floor structures ensure normal function of the urethra.[16–18] The signs and symptoms of pelvic floor dysfunction often overlap with signs and symptoms of urethral diverticula, ectopic ureters, urethral tumors, and periurethral cystic lesions. Ectopic ureters and ureteroceles are usually diagnosed in childhood and rarely present in adults. Nevertheless, these conditions should be considered in patients with urinary tract infections or urinary incontinence because surgery can correct these disorders.[19] Endovaginal ultrasound is a useful tool in the diagnosis of ectopic and dystopic ureters.[20] Urethral diverticula are also occasionally found in women complaining of urinary incontinence and/or pain and dyspareunia. Ultrasound can help differentiate a diverticulum from other periurethral cystic lesions, such as ectopic ureters, calcifications, and injected material, and is useful in surgical planning because it can offer invaluable information, such as shape, size, and location in relation to the urethra and bladder.[21] Endovaginal ultrasound is very useful in the diagnosis and monitoring of urethral tumors.[22] An example is a urethral leiomyoma, which is a rare benign smooth muscle tumor that may grow in pregnancy and cause dysuria. On ultrasound these tumors appear well defined, homogenous, with increased vascularity.[23] Urethral carcinoma is a rare cancer that accounts for less than 0.02% of all malignancies in women and typically appears as an anterior urethral tumor.[23] Endovaginal ultrasound of the bladder can provide important information regarding the bladder neck, and the diagnosis of foreign bodies and bladder diverticula. Bladder wall thickness can also be measured by endovaginal ultrasound and has been found to positively correlate with detrusor instability.[24]

Central Compartment

Assessment of the central compartment is usually performed with transperineal ultrasound. Endovaginal techniques have a limited role in assessing the central compartment because the probe impedes descent of the uterus or vault. Additionally uterine or vaginal vault prolapse is typically diagnosed on clinical examination.

Posterior Compartment

For the posterior compartment, endovaginal ultrasound with a biplane transducer provides important information including ensuring integrity of the rectovaginal septum, and measuring the anorectal angle. During Valsalva, several other important aspects are appreciated including descent of an enterocele, rectocele, and movement of the puborectalis and anorectal angle to evaluate for pelvic floor dyssynergy, and visualization of intussusception.[9] Transvaginal 3D ultrasound also is a useful tool in visualizing rectovaginal fistulae.[25] Assessment of the anal canal is typically performed with endoanal ultrasound (discussed later).[11,26]

The anatomic causes associated with defecatory dysfunction are best visualized on dynamic transperineal or translabial and endovaginal scans.[27] Many clinicians use the term "rectocele" to refer to any prolapse of the posterior vaginal wall; a true rectocele is defined as herniation of the anterior rectal wall into the vagina.[28] Although examination is usually adequate to diagnose prolapse of the posterior vaginal wall, ultrasound is a useful tool in diagnosing a true rectocele. Typically this is done with a transperineal ultrasound because the endoluminal ultrasound probe may prevent the prolapse from occurring.

An enterocele is a hernia of the most inferior point of the abdominal cavity into the vagina or pouch of Douglas. On ultrasound, it is visualized as the downward movement of abdominal contents into the vagina, ventral to the rectal ampulla and anal canal. A sigmoidocele can usually be seen by differentiating hyperechoic stool movement from the surrounding tissue. Being able to differentiate a sigmoidocele from an enterocele is important in planning a surgical procedure. By definition, an intussusception occurs when the rectal wall telescopes into the rectal lumen and may involve the rectal mucosa or full thickness of the rectal wall. It is defined as intra-rectal, intra-anal, or external if it forms a complete rectal prolapse. Pelvic floor dyssynergy is typically described as a lack of normal relaxation of the puborectalis muscle during defecation. This is a difficult condition to verify through clinical examination. However, during Valsalva, it is documented by ultrasound because the anorectal angle becomes narrower, the levator hiatus is shortened, and the puborectalis muscle thickens.[27]

Lateral Compartments

Until recently, the concept of pelvic floor trauma focused mainly on perineal, vaginal, and anal sphincter injuries. But over the past several years, with advancements of 3D ultrasound technology, the concept of levator ani injury has become an important component of pelvic floor trauma. The pelvic floor is composed of symmetrically paired levator ani muscles, which together form a sheet of muscles attached to the internal surface of the true pelvis. The levator ani is divided into three muscle groups, named for their attachments: (1) pubovisceralis, (2) puborectalis, and (3) iliococcygeus. The pubovisceralis is further divided into the puboperinealis, pubovaginalis, and puboanalis muscles.[29] Together, these muscles support the urogenital organs and the anorectum.

Studies have shown that levator ani injury is common. Levator avulsion is the disconnection of the levator ani from its insertion on the pubic ramus or pelvic sidewall. Levator tears can occur at any part of the muscle between the two insertion points. Avulsion and tears are a common complication of overstretching of the muscles during childbirth and occur in 10% to 36% of women in their first vaginal delivery.[28,30–32] Not only can childbirth injure the muscles of the pelvic floor, but it can also disrupt the innervation of the muscles.[33] Electromyography abnormalities in the pelvic floor associated with defecation disorders, stress urinary incontinence, and prolapse are more frequently seen in women who are multiparous, who have had prolonged second stages of labor, forceps delivery, and high birth weight.[34–37]

Levator ani injury has been shown to be negatively correlated with pelvic floor strength, and positively correlated with fecal incontinence and stage of pelvic organ prolapse. Steensma and colleagues[38] found that weak pelvic floor muscles occurred more often in women who had levator ani avulsion, with injuries being present in 53.8% of women with weak pelvic floor strength compared with being present in 16.1% of women with normal strength. Women with levator ani injury have been found to have a greater incidence of fecal incontinence.[39] Particularly the puborectalis muscle plays an important role in maintaining continence, as shown in a case-control study that found that fecal incontinence was more common in women with puborectalis abnormalities compared with control subjects.[40] It is well established that women with levator ani injury have a higher risk of developing pelvic organ prolapse.[41] Levator avulsion seems to play a significant role particularly in the central and anterior compartments because the risk of having prolapse in these compartments doubles with levator ani avulsion.[42] The relationship with stress incontinence and levator ani injury is unclear because some studies shown no correlation,[43] whereas others have shown a negative correlation.[44] However, women with previous stress incontinence are twice as likely to have a levator ani injury during childbirth.[45]

Levator avulsion can be accurately seen through 3D endovaginal ultrasound imaging, especially during a pelvic floor muscle contraction. Because levator damage from childbirth is not always an "all or none" phenomenon, a scoring system was developed to quantify levator ani injury with 3D endovaginal ultrasound. This scoring system has been shown to have high interrater reliability.[46,47]

Implanted Vaginal Material

Over the last two decades, pelvic floor surgeries involving permanent vagina implants used to aid in pelvic organ prolapse and stress incontinence have risen in popularity. Polypropylene mesh is one of the most commonly used meshes in vaginal surgery and is highly echogenic on endovaginal ultrasound. Imaging can determine the size, shape, position, distortion, and mobility of the implants. Position of the mesh is typically either along the posterior vaginal wall sometimes extending to the perineal body, along the anterior wall, or near the midurethra in the case of midurethral slings. Often the implanted mesh is found to be shrunken, contracted, or folded.[48] **Fig. 3** shows an example of anterior and posterior vaginal wall mesh materials. In the case of midurethral slings, ultrasound can help distinguish transobturator versus retropubic slings, and help locate and map the location of the synthetic material on axial imaging of the anterior compartment relative to the bladder neck.[49,50] **Fig. 4** shows an example of a transobturator sling visualized on ultrasound. This is helpful in planning a procedure to remove permanent synthetic materials in the absence of an operative report, or as adjunctive imaging in cases where the synthetic materials appear displaced. Periurethral bulking agents can also easily be seen on endovaginal ultrasound.[50]

Endoanal Imaging

Endoanal ultrasound is the gold standard for morphologic assessment of the anal canal.[11] When performing endoanal ultrasound, the anal canal is divided into three levels in the axial plan: (1) upper, (2) middle, and (3) lower.[9] The uppermost level is marked proximally by the puborectalis muscle and distally by the ring of the IAS. The middle level is marked by the complete ring of the IAS and EAS, and the visualization of the

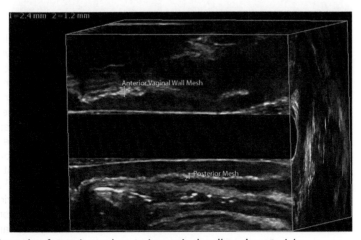

Fig. 3. Example of anterior and posterior vaginal wall mesh materials.

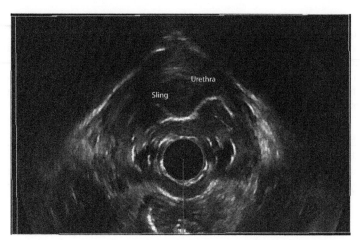

Fig. 4. Example of a transobturator sling visualized on ultrasound.

transverse perinei muscles. The lower level is marked by the subcutaneous part of the EAS. **Fig. 5** shows an example of normal IAS and EAS anatomy.

Endoanal ultrasound is often the diagnostic test of choice in patients presenting with fecal incontinence and a history of a traumatic childbirth. **Fig. 6** shows an example of a combined IAS and EAS defect. Fecal incontinence is defined as the involuntary loss of feces, whereas anal incontinence is the involuntary loss of flatus or feces. It is an embarrassing problem that has a devastating impact on a woman's life. Because of the embarrassing nature of the problem, women often do not complain to their physician, making the true incidence of anal incontinence likely underestimated. Reported prevalence varies widely, ranging from 1% to 24% of the US adult population, and is projected to increase 59% by 2050.[51–57] An intact, innervated, and well-functioning

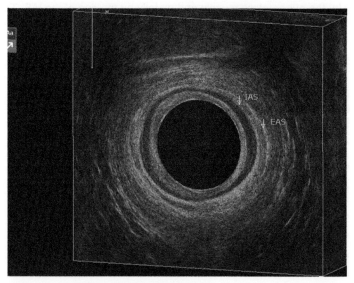

Fig. 5. Example of normal IAS and EAS anatomy.

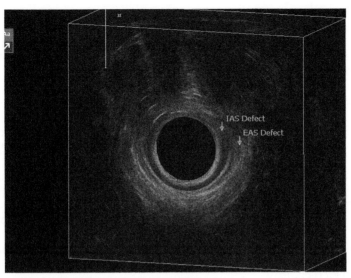

Fig. 6. Example of a combined IAS and EAS defect.

IAS, EAS, and puborectalis muscle is a prerequisite for fecal control. Anal sphincter defects most often occur following instrumented vaginal deliveries, and are a common cause of fecal incontinence. Sultan and colleagues[58] found in a study of 79 primiparous women that 35% of them had defects of either the IAS or the EAS or both 6 weeks after delivery. Forceps-assisted vaginal deliveries are associated with 80% chance of having sphincter defects found after delivery[58] and a 32% chance of having anal incontinence.[59] Endoanal ultrasound has been found to be superior to other diagnostic tools for the evaluation of sphincter defects with a sensitivity of 100%, compared with a sensitivity of 89% for electromyography, 67% for manometry, and 57% for clinical assessment.[60] When performing anal ultrasonography the EAS appears hyperechoic and has a heterogeneous appearance, whereas the IAS appears homogeneously hypoechoic. By defining the margins of disruption, it provides invaluable information for the surgeon if surgical repair is considered.

Surgical repair of hemorrhoids, anal fissures, and anal fistulas can also be a cause of anal sphincter disruption leading to fecal and anal incontinence. Hemorrhoids cause soiling and endoanal ultrasound can be particularly useful in diagnosing internal hemorrhoids. However, surgical excision of internal hemorrhoids can lead to damage of the IAS and anal incontinence.[61] Hemorrhoid stapling has been shown to prevent IAS damage as opposed to hemorrhoid excision.[62] An anal stretch procedure, done for anal fissures, is associated with a 27% chance of anal incontinence after the procedure with 90% of those patients having evidence of IAS disruption on endoanal ultrasound.[63] Although endoanal ultrasound is helpful in diagnosing fistula tracts involving the anus and rectum, it can also be useful in diagnosing anal sphincter injury after surgical correction of the fistula.[64]

SUMMARY

This article provides a background and appraisal of endoluminal ultrasound of the pelvic floor. It offers a detailed anatomic assessment of the muscles and surrounding organs of the pelvic floor. Different anatomic variability and pathology, such as prolapse, fecal incontinence, urinary incontinence, vaginal wall cysts, synthetic implanted material, and pelvic pain, are easily assessed with endoluminal vaginal ultrasound. With pelvic organ prolapse in particular, not only is the prolapse itself seen but the underlying cause related to the anatomic and functional abnormalities of the pelvic floor muscle structures are also visualized.

REFERENCES

1. Dietz HP, Hyland G, Hay-Smith J. The assessment of levator trauma: a comparison between palpation and 4D pelvic floor ultrasound. Neurourol Urodyn 2006; 25(5):424–7.
2. Kearney R, Miller JM, Delancey JO. Interrater reliability and physical examination of the pubovisceral portion of the levator ani muscle, validity comparisons using MR imaging. Neurourol Urodyn 2006;25(1):50–4.
3. Dietz HP, Shek C. Validity and reproducibility of the digital detection of levator trauma. Int Urogynecol J Pelvic Floor Dysfunct 2008;19(8):1097–101.
4. Shobeiri SA, Leclaire E, Nihira MA, et al. Appearance of the levator ani muscle subdivisions in endovaginal three-dimensional ultrasonography. Obstet Gynecol 2009;114(1):66–72.
5. Margulies RU, Hsu Y, Kearney R, et al. Appearance of the levator ani muscle subdivisions in magnetic resonance images. Obstet Gynecol 2006;107(5):1064–9.
6. Lien KC, Mooney B, DeLancey JO, et al. Levator ani muscle stretch induced by simulated vaginal birth. Obstet Gynecol 2004;103(1):31–40.
7. Dietz HP. Pelvic floor ultrasound: a review. Am J Obstet Gynecol 2010;202(4): 321–34.
8. Dietz HP. Ultrasound imaging of the pelvic floor. Part II: three-dimensional or volume imaging. Ultrasound Obstet Gynecol 2004;23(6):615–25.
9. Santoro GA, Wieczorek AP, Dietz HP, et al. State of the art: an integrated approach to pelvic floor ultrasonography. Ultrasound Obstet Gynecol 2011; 37(4):381–96.
10. Santoro GA, Wieczorek AP, Stankiewicz A, et al. High-resolution three-dimensional endovaginal ultrasonography in the assessment of pelvic floor anatomy: a preliminary study. Int Urogynecol J Pelvic Floor Dysfunct 2009;20(10):1213–22.
11. Abdool Z, Sultan AH, Thakar R. Ultrasound imaging of the anal sphincter complex: a review. Br J Radiol 2012;85(1015):865–75.
12. Thakar R, Sultan AH. Anal endosonography and its role in assessing the incontinent patient. Best Pract Res Clin Obstet Gynaecol 2004;18(1):157–73.
13. Dietz HP, Haylen BT, Vancaillie TG. Female pelvic organ prolapse and voiding function. Int Urogynecol J Pelvic Floor Dysfunct 2002;13(5):284–8.
14. Shobeiri SA, White D, Quiroz LH, et al. Anterior and posterior compartment 3D endovaginal ultrasound anatomy based on direct histologic comparison. Int Urogynecol J 2012;23(8):1047–53.
15. Shobeiri SA, Rostaminia G, White D, et al. Evaluation of vaginal cysts and masses by 3-dimensional endovaginal and endoanal sonography. J Ultrasound Med 2013;32(8):1499–507.
16. Petros PE, Ulmsten UI. An integral theory and its method for the diagnosis and management of female urinary incontinence. Scand J Urol Nephrol Suppl 1993; 153:1–93.
17. Petros PE, Ulmsten UI. An integral theory of female urinary incontinence. Experimental and clinical considerations. Acta Obstet Gynecol Scand Suppl 1990;153: 7–31.

18. Petros PE, Woodman PJ. The integral theory of continence. Int Urogynecol J Pelvic Floor Dysfunct 2008;19(1):35–40.
19. Wang S, Lang JH, Zhou HM. Symptomatic urinary problems in female genital tract anomalies. Int Urogynecol J Pelvic Floor Dysfunct 2009;20(4):401–6.
20. Yang JM, Huang WC, Yang SH. Transvaginal sonography in the diagnosis, management and follow-up of complex paraurethral abnormalities. Ultrasound Obstet Gynecol 2005;25(3):302–6.
21. Chaudhari VV, Patel MK, Douek M, et al. MR imaging and US of female urethral and periurethral disease. Radiographics 2010;30(7):1857–74.
22. Yang JM, Yang SH, Huang WC. Two- and three-dimensional sonographic findings in a case of distal urethral obstruction due to a paraurethral tumor. Ultrasound Obstet Gynecol 2005;25(5):519–21.
23. Shobeiri SA. Practical pelvic floor ultrasonography, a multicompartmental approach to 2D/3D/4D ultrasonography of pelvic floor. New York: Springer; 2013.
24. Khullar V, Salvatore S, Cardozo L, et al. A novel technique for measuring bladder wall thickness in women using transvaginal ultrasound. Ultrasound Obstet Gynecol 1994;4(3):220–3.
25. Denson L, Shobeiri SA. Peroxide-enhanced 3-dimensional endovaginal ultrasound imaging for diagnosis of rectovaginal fistula. Female Pelvic Med Reconstr Surg 2014;20(4):240–2.
26. Santoro GA, Fortling B. The advantages of volume rendering in three-dimensional endosonography of the anorectum. Dis Colon Rectum 2007;50(3):359–68.
27. Santiago AC, O'Leary DE, Quiroz LH, et al. An ultrasound approach to the posterior compartment and anorectal dysfunction. Int Urogynecol J 2015;26(9):1393–4.
28. Dietz HP, Moegni F, Shek KL. Diagnosis of levator avulsion injury: a comparison of three methods. Ultrasound Obstet Gynecol 2012;40(6):693–8.
29. Kearney R, Sawhney R, DeLancey JO. Levator ani muscle anatomy evaluated by origin-insertion pairs. Obstet Gynecol 2004;104(1):168–73.
30. Dietz HP, Lanzarone V. Levator trauma after vaginal delivery. Obstet Gynecol 2005;106(4):707–12.
31. Chan SS, Cheung RY, Yiu KW, et al. Pelvic floor biometry in Chinese primiparous women 1 year after delivery: a prospective observational study. Ultrasound Obstet Gynecol 2014;43(4):466–74.
32. Shek KL, Dietz HP. The effect of childbirth on hiatal dimensions. Obstet Gynecol 2009;113(6):1272–8.
33. South MM, Stinnett SS, Sanders DB, et al. Levator ani denervation and reinnervation 6 months after childbirth. Am J Obstet Gynecol 2009;200(5):519.e1–7.
34. Snooks SJ, Henry MM, Swash M. Faecal incontinence due to external anal sphincter division in childbirth is associated with damage to the innervation of the pelvic floor musculature: a double pathology. Br J Obstet Gynaecol 1985;92(8):824–8.
35. Snooks SJ, Setchell M, Swash M, et al. Injury to innervation of pelvic floor sphincter musculature in childbirth. Lancet 1984;2(8402):546–50.
36. Weidner AC, Jamison MG, Branham V, et al. Neuropathic injury to the levator ani occurs in 1 in 4 primiparous women. Am J Obstet Gynecol 2006;195(6):1851–6.
37. Allen RE, Hosker GL, Smith AR, et al. Pelvic floor damage and childbirth: a neurophysiological study. Br J Obstet Gynaecol 1990;97(9):770–9.
38. Steensma AB, Konstantinovic ML, Burger CW, et al. Prevalence of major levator abnormalities in symptomatic patients with an underactive pelvic floor contraction. Int Urogynecol J 2010;21(7):861–7.

39. Heilbrun ME, Nygaard IE, Lockhart ME, et al. Correlation between levator ani muscle injuries on magnetic resonance imaging and fecal incontinence, pelvic organ prolapse, and urinary incontinence in primiparous women. Am J Obstet Gynecol 2010;202(5):488.e1–6.

40. Weinstein MM, Pretorius DH, Jung SA, et al. Transperineal three-dimensional ultrasound imaging for detection of anatomic defects in the anal sphincter complex muscles. Clin Gastroenterol Hepatol 2009;7(2):205–11.

41. DeLancey JO, Morgan DM, Fenner DE, et al. Comparison of levator ani muscle defects and function in women with and without pelvic organ prolapse. Obstet Gynecol 2007;109(2 Pt 1):295–302.

42. Dietz HP. Quantification of major morphological abnormalities of the levator ani. Ultrasound Obstet Gynecol 2007;29(3):329–34.

43. DeLancey JO, Trowbridge ER, Miller JM, et al. Stress urinary incontinence: relative importance of urethral support and urethral closure pressure. J Urol 2008; 179(6):2286–90 [discussion: 2290].

44. Dietz HP, Kirby A. Modelling the likelihood of levator avulsion in a urogynaecological population. Aust N Z J Obstet Gynaecol 2010;50(3):268–72.

45. DeLancey JO, Kearney R, Chou Q, et al. The appearance of levator ani muscle abnormalities in magnetic resonance images after vaginal delivery. Obstet Gynecol 2003;101(1):46–53.

46. Rostaminia G, Manonai J, Leclaire E, et al. Interrater reliability of assessing levator ani deficiency with 360 degrees 3D endovaginal ultrasound. Int Urogynecol J 2014;25(6):761–6.

47. Rostaminia G, White D, Hegde A, et al. Levator ani deficiency and pelvic organ prolapse severity. Obstet Gynecol 2013;121(5):1017–24.

48. Tunn R, Picot A, Marschke J, et al. Sonomorphological evaluation of polypropylene mesh implants after vaginal mesh repair in women with cystocele or rectocele. Ultrasound Obstet Gynecol 2007;29(4):449–52.

49. Dietz HP, Barry C, Lim YN, et al. Two-dimensional and three-dimensional ultrasound imaging of suburethral slings. Ultrasound Obstet Gynecol 2005;26(2):175–9.

50. Denson L, Shobeiri SA. Three-dimensional endovaginal sonography of synthetic implanted materials in the female pelvic floor. J Ultrasound Med 2014;33(3):521–9.

51. Drossman DA, Li Z, Andruzzi E, et al. U.S. householder survey of functional gastrointestinal disorders. Prevalence, sociodemography, and health impact. Dig Dis Sci 1993;38(9):1569–80.

52. Macmillan AK, Merrie AE, Marshall RJ, et al. The prevalence of fecal incontinence in community-dwelling adults: a systematic review of the literature. Dis Colon Rectum 2004;47(8):1341–9.

53. Markland AD, Goode PS, Burgio KL, et al. Incidence and risk factors for fecal incontinence in black and white older adults: a population-based study. J Am Geriatr Soc 2010;58(7):1341–6.

54. Nelson R, Norton N, Cautley E, et al. Community-based prevalence of anal incontinence. JAMA 1995;274(7):559–61.

55. Varma MG, Brown JS, Creasman JM, et al. Fecal incontinence in females older than aged 40 years: who is at risk? Dis Colon Rectum 2006;49(6):841–51.

56. Whitehead WE, Borrud L, Goode PS, et al. Fecal incontinence in US adults: epidemiology and risk factors. Gastroenterology 2009;137(2):512–7, 512.e1–2.

57. Wu JM, Vaughan CP, Goode PS, et al. Prevalence and trends of symptomatic pelvic floor disorders in U.S. women. Obstet Gynecol 2014;123(1):141–8.

58. Sultan AH, Kamm MA, Hudson CN, et al. Anal-sphincter disruption during vaginal delivery. N Engl J Med 1993;329(26):1905–11.
59. Sultan AH, Johanson RB, Carter JE. Occult anal sphincter trauma following randomized forceps and vacuum delivery. Int J Gynaecol Obstet 1998;61(2):113–9.
60. Sultan AH, Nicholls RJ, Kamm MA, et al. Anal endosonography and correlation with in vitro and in vivo anatomy. Br J Surg 1993;80(4):508–11.
61. Speakman CT, Burnett SJ, Kamm MA, et al. Sphincter injury after anal dilatation demonstrated by anal endosonography. Br J Surg 1991;78(12):1429–30.
62. Altomare DF, Rinaldi M, Sallustio PL, et al. Long-term effects of stapled haemorrhoidectomy on internal anal function and sensitivity. Br J Surg 2001;88(11): 1487–91.
63. Khubchandani IT, Reed JF. Sequelae of internal sphincterotomy for chronic fissure in ano. Br J Surg 1989;76(5):431–4.
64. Kennedy HL, Zegarra JP. Fistulotomy without external sphincter division for high anal fistulae. Br J Surg 1990;77(8):898–901.

Index

Note: Page numbers of article titles are in **boldface** type.

Obstet Gynecol Clin N Am 43 (2016) 155–164
http://dx.doi.org/10.1016/S0889-8545(16)00009-7
0889-8545/16/$ – see front matter © 2016 Elsevier Inc. All rights reserved.

obgyn.theclinics.com

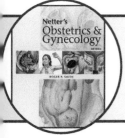

Moving?

Make sure your subscription moves with you!

To notify us of your new address, find your **Clinics Account Number** (located on your mailing label above your name), and contact customer service at:

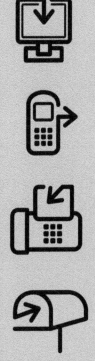

Email: journalscustomerservice-usa@elsevier.com

800-654-2452 (subscribers in the U.S. & Canada)
314-447-8871 (subscribers outside of the U.S. & Canada)

Fax number: 314-447-8029

Elsevier Health Sciences Division
Subscription Customer Service
3251 Riverport Lane
Maryland Heights, MO 63043

Printed and bound by CPI Group (UK) Ltd, Croydon, CR0 4YY

07/10/2024

01040498-0016